Rapid Obstetrics & Gynaecology

Misha Moore
MBChB BSc MPH MRCOG

Sarah-Jane Lam
MBBS MA (cantab) MRCOG

Adam R Kay
MBBS

All Registrars in Obstetrics and Gynaecology, London Deanery

Second Edition

WILEY-BLACKWELL
A Blackwell Publishing Ltd., Publication

This edition first published 2010, © 2010 by Misha Moore, Sarah-Jane Lam and Adam R Kay
Previous edition published 2004

Blackwell Publishing was acquired by John Wiley & Sons in February 2007. Blackwell's publishing program has been merged with Wiley's global Scientific, Technical and Medical business to form Wiley-Blackwell.

Registered office: John Wiley & Sons Ltd, The Atrium, Southern Gate, Chichester, West Sussex, PO19 8SQ, UK

Editorial offices: 9600 Garsington Road, Oxford, OX4 2DQ, UK
                          The Atrium, Southern Gate, Chichester, West Sussex, PO19 8SQ, UK
                          111 River Street, Hoboken, NJ 07030-5774, USA

For details of our global editorial offices, for customer services and for information about how to apply for permission to reuse the copyright material in this book please see our website at www.wiley.com/wiley-blackwell

Library of Congress Cataloging-in-Publication Data

Rapid obstetrics & gynaecology / Misha Moore, Sarah Jane Lam, Adam R. Kay. – 2nd ed.
        p. ; cm. – (Rapid series)
  Other title: Rapid obstetrics and gynaecology
  ISBN 978-1-4051-9450-1
  1. Obstetrics–Handbooks, manuals, etc. 2. Gynecology–Handbooks, manuals, etc. I. Moore, Misha. II. Lam, Sarah Jane. III. Kay, Adam R. IV. Title: Rapid obstetrics and gynaecology. V. Series: Rapid series.
  [DNLM: 1. Genital Diseases, Female–Handbooks. 2. Gynecology–Handbooks. 3. Obstetrics–Handbooks. 4. Pregnancy Complications–Handbooks. WQ 39 R218 2010]
  RG110.R37 2010
  618–dc22

                                        2010010782

ISBN: 9781405194501

A catalogue record for this book is available from the British Library.

Set in 7.5/9.5pt Frutiger-Light by Thomson Digital, Noida, India

Printed and bound in Malaysia by Vivar Printing Sdn Bhd

1   2010

Contents

Gynaecology

Procedures

Appendices

Preface

Obstetrics and Gynaecology can be a bewildering new world for both undergraduates and new trainees. Despite your wealth of clinical exposure you can find yourself back to square one, surrounded by brand new diseases and the mystifying territory of the Labour Ward.

The simple and structured nature of *Rapid Obstetrics and Gynaecology* lends itself extremely well to tackling the subject. By identifying the *key topics*, and distilling from these the *key facts*, this book will provide you with firm foundations and we hope to encourage some of you into this most rewarding of specialties.

MM, SJL, ARK
2010

List of abbreviations

ABC	airway, breathing, circulation
ABG	arterial blood gas
ACE	angiotensin-converting enzyme
ACTH	adrenocorticotrophic hormone
AFP	alphafetoprotein
AIDS	acquired immune deficiency syndrome
AIS	androgen insensitivity syndrome
AMA	anti-mitochondrial antibodies
APH	antepartum haemorrhage
ARDS	acute respiratory distress syndrome
ARM	artificial rupture of membranes
ASMA	anti-smooth muscle antibodies
ASD	atrial septal defect
BMI	body mass index
BP	blood pressure
bpm	beats per minute
BSO	bilateral salpingo-oophorectomy
BV	bacterial vaginosis
CAH	congenital adrenal hyperplasia
CBT	cognitive behavioural therapy
CEA	carcinoembryonic antigen
CMV	cytomegalovirus
CNS	central nervous system
COCP	combined oral contraceptive pill
CPD	cephalopelvic disproportion
CT	computerised tomography
CTPA	computerised tomography pulmonary angiogram
CTG	cardiotocograph
CVA	cerebrovascular accident
CVP	central venous pressure
CVS	chorionic villous sampling
CXR	chest x-ray
D&E	dilatation and evacuation
DIC	disseminated intravascular coagulation
DVT	deep vein thrombosis
EBV	Epstein–Barr virus
ECG	electrocardiogram
echo	echocardiogram
ECT	electroconvulsive therapy
ECV	external cephalic version
ERPC	evacuation of retained products of conception
FBC	full blood count
FBS	fetal blood sampling
FEV	forced expiratory volume
FFP	fresh frozen plasma
FH	fetal heart
FHR	fetal heart rate
FSE	fetal scalp electrode
FSH	follicle stimulating hormone
FTA-ABS	fluorescent treponemal antibody absorption

GBS	group B Streptococcus
GDM	gestational diabetes mellitus
GFR	glomerular filtration rate
GGT	gamma glutamyl transferase
GnRH	gonadotrophin-releasing hormone
GTT	glucose tolerance test
G&S	group and save
HAART	highly active antiretroviral therapy
HbA1c	glycosylated haemoglobin
HBsAg	hepatitis B surface antigen
HCG	human chorionic gonadotrophin
HG	hyperemesis gravidarum
HNPCC	hereditary non-polyposis colon cancer
HELLP	haemolysis, elevated liver enzymes, low platelets
HIV	human immunodeficiency virus
HPL	human placental lactogen
HPV	human papilloma virus
HR	heart rate
HRT	hormone replacement therapy
HSG	hysterosalpingogram
HSV	herpes simplex virus
HVS	high vaginal swab
ICSI	intracytoplasmic sperm injection
IM	intramuscular
IOL	induction of labour
IMB	intermenstrual bleeding
IPPV	intermittent positive-pressure ventilation
ITP	idiopathic thrombocytopenic purpura
ITU	intensive treatment unit
IUCD	intrauterine contraceptive device
IUD	intrauterine death
IUGR	intrauterine growth restriction
IUS	intrauterine system (contains levonorgestrel)
IUI	intrauterine insemination
IV	intravenous
IVF	in-vitro infertilisation
JVP	jugular venous pressure
LFD	large for dates
LFT	liver function tests
LH	luteinising hormone
LLETZ	large loop excision of the transformation zone
LMP	last menstrual period
LMWH	low molecular weight heparin
LVEF	left ventricular ejection fraction
LVF	left ventricular failure
LVS	low vaginal swab
MC&S	microscopy culture and sensitivity
MCV	mean corpuscular volume
$MgSO_4$	magnesium sulphate
MMR	measles, mumps, rubella vaccine
MRI	magnetic resonance imaging
MS	multiple sclerosis
MSU	mid-stream urine
NSAIDS	non-steroidal anti-inflammatory drugs

NT	nuchal translucency
OA	occipitoanterior
OHSS	ovarian hyperstimulation syndrome
OT	occipitotransverse
OP	occipitoposterior
PAPP-A	pregnancy-associated plasma protein A
PCB	postcoital bleeding
PCOS	polycystic ovarian syndrome
PCR	polymerase chain reaction
PDA	patent ductus arteriosus
PE	pulmonary embolism
PEFR	peak expiratory flow rate
PET	pre-eclamptic toxaemia
PID	pelvic inflammatory disease
PMB	postmenopausal bleeding
PO	by mouth
POP	progesterone-only pill
PPH	postpartum haemorrhage
PPROM	pre-term premature rupture of membranes
PR	per rectum
PROM	prelabour rupture of membranes
PTL	preterm labour
PV	per vagina
RhD	Rhesus D antigen
RMC	recurrent miscarriage
RPOC	retained products of conception
RPR	rapid plasma reagin
SC	subcuticular
SERMs	selective (o)estrogen receptor modulators
SFD	small for dates
SHBG	sex-hormone binding globulin
SLE	systemic lupus erythematosus
SROM	spontaneous rupture of membranes
SSRI	selective serotonin reuptake inhibitor
STI	sexually transmitted infection
TAH	total abdominal hysterectomy
TFT	thyroid function tests
TOP	termination of pregnancy
TORCH	toxoplasma rubella cytomegalovirus herpes simplex
TPHA	Treponema pallidum haemagglutination assay
TSH	thyroid stimulating hormone
TTTS	twin-to-twin transfusion syndrome
TVS	transvaginal scan
TVT	tension-free vaginal tape
U&E	urea and electrolytes
USS	ultrasound scan
UTI	urinary tract infection
VDRL	Venereal Disease Research Laboratory
VIN	vaginal intraepithelial neoplasia
V/Q	ventilation perfusion (scan)
VSD	ventricular septal defect
VTE	venous thromboembolism
VZIG	varicella zoster immunoglobulin
X-match	crossmatch

Obstetrics

Acute fatty liver of pregnancy

DEFINITION Rare pregnancy-associated disorder characterised by fatty infiltration of the liver.

AETIOLOGY Likely to be due to a mitochondrial disorder affecting fatty acid oxidation.

ASSOCIATIONS/RISK FACTORS Nulliparity, multiple pregnancy, obesity, male fetus, pre-eclampsia.

EPIDEMIOLOGY UK prevalence estimated at 5 per 100 000.

HISTORY Often non-specific, normally in third trimester: nausea, vomiting, abdominal pain, jaundice, bleeding.

EXAMINATION Liver tenderness, jaundice, ascites, manifestations of coagulopathy. Fifty percent of women will have proteinuric hypertension.

PATHOLOGY/PATHOGENESIS Accumulation of microvesicular fat in haepatocytes, periportal sparing, small yellow liver on gross examination.

INVESTIGATIONS

Bloods: FBC (assess Hb, haemoconcentration, thrombocytopenia), clotting ($\downarrow$ synthesis + consumption of clotting factors), LFT ($\uparrow$ transaminases, mild hyperbilirubinaemia), U&E, glucose (hypoglycaemia common).

MANAGEMENT Delivery is necessary to halt deterioration. Treatment is supportive: fluid management; correction of hypoglycaemia; blood transfusion as appropriate; correction of coagulopathy with platelets/FFP/cryoprecipitate. Liver transplantation is rarely necessary.

COMPLICATIONS

Maternal: Death, haemorrhage (secondary to DIC), renal failure, hepatic encephalopathy, sepsis, pancreatitis.
Fetal: Death.

PROGNOSIS Maternal mortality 10–20%; perinatal mortality 20–30%.

Amniotic fluid embolism

DEFINITION Obstetric emergency in which amniotic fluid and fetal cells enter the maternal circulation causing cardiorespiratory collapse.

AETIOLOGY Unclear. Entry of amniotic fluid or fetal debris to the maternal circulation provokes either an anaphylactoid reaction or activation of the complement cascade.

ASSOCIATIONS/RISK FACTORS Often occurs in the absence of identifiable risk factors. Multiparity, ↑ maternal age, Caesarean section, uterine hyperstimulation, use of uterotonics, placental abruption, trauma, termination of pregnancy.

EPIDEMIOLOGY UK prevalence is 1.8 per 100 000 maternities.

HISTORY Sudden-onset dyspnoea ± chest pain, ?collapse.

EXAMINATION Tachypneoa, cyanosis, hypotension, tachycardia, evidence of coagulopathy.

PATHOLOGY/PATHOGENESIS The precipitating reaction causes pulmonary artery spasm, ↑ pulmonary arterial pressure and ↑ right ventricular pressure, resulting in hypoxia. Hypoxia leads to myocardial and pulmonary capillary damage and LVF. Post mortem reveals fetal squames and debris in the maternal pulmonary circulation.

INVESTIGATIONS
Bloods: ABG, FBC, clotting, U&E, X-match.
Imaging: CXR.
Other: ECG.

MANAGEMENT Largely supportive; manage in ITU.
Airway: Maintain patency.
Breathing: High-flow oxygen ± intubation.
Circulation: Two large-bore IV cannulae, fluid resuscitation, consider pulmonary artery catheter and ionotropic support, correct coagulopathy with FFP/cryoprecipitate/platelets, blood transfusion if necessary.

Consider delivery.

COMPLICATIONS Cardiac arrest, death, DIC, seizures, uterine atony and haemorrhage, pulmonary oedema, ARDS, renal failure.

PROGNOSIS In the UK: 37% mortality, of which 25% occurs within the first hour.

Cardiac disease in pregnancy

DEFINITION Cardiac disease in a pregnant woman.

AETIOLOGY

Congenital heart disease: PDA, ASD, VSD, coarctation of the aorta, Marfan's, Fallot's tetralogy, Eisenmenger's syndrome.

Acquired heart disease: Valvular defects, ischaemic heart disease.

Cardomyopathies: Including peripartum cardiomyopathy (new-onset cardiomyopathy and heart failure usually within time period of last month of pregnancy and 5 months post-partum).

ASSOCIATIONS/RISK FACTORS As for cardiac disease in general: family history, obesity, hypertension, smoking, ↑ age, diabetes.

EPIDEMIOLOGY Increasing prevalence due to ↑ maternal age, ↑ life expectancy for patients with congenital heart disease, ↑ immigrant populations.

HISTORY Assess new/deterioration of symptoms: SOB, palpitations, orthopnoea, paroxysmal nocturnal dyspnoea, decreased exercise tolerance, chest pain.

EXAMINATION

General: Pulse, BP, JVP, ?oedema, ?cyanosis.

Chest: Heart sounds, murmurs (*note:* ejection systolic common in pregnancy), basal crepitations.

Abdomen: Fundal height (associated with IUGR).

PATHOLOGY/PATHOGENESIS Dependent on aetiologies noted above. There is 40% increase in blood volume during pregnancy, hence cardiac strain. Women with cardiac disease are unable to increase cardiac output (uterine hypoperfusion, ↑risk of pulmonary oedema).

INVESTIGATIONS

Bloods: FBC, U&E, LFT.

Cardiac: ECG, echo.

Fetus: Serial USS for fetal growth, cardiac anomaly scan if there is maternal congenital heart disease.

MANAGEMENT Dependent on the aetiology.

General: Combined obstetric/cardiology care (tertiary referral centre).

Preconceptual: Assess cardiac status, address risks and absolute contraindications to pregnancy.

Antenatal: Optimise treatment, monitor fetal wellbeing, consider thromboprophylaxis.

Delivery: Consider optimum mode and timing of delivery, consult with anaesthetists, correct positioning, fluid management, consider antibiotic prophylaxis (structural defects).

Post-partum: Increase surveillance (period of haemodynamic change).

COMPLICATIONS

Maternal: Progression of disease, VTE, pulmonary oedema, death.

Fetal: PTL, ↑ congenital heart disease (if maternal congenital heart disease), IUGR, effects of teratogenic drugs for anticoagulation, fetal death.

PROGNOSIS High risk of maternal mortality if LVEF <40% or LVF. Pulmonary hypertension: 20–50% maternal mortality rate. Eisenmenger's: 50% maternal mortality rate. Patients with Marfan's syndrome with aortic root >4–4.5 cm are advised against pregnancy.

Chronic hypertension in pregnancy

DEFINITION Hypertension that is either present prior to conception (detected before 20/40) or persists after pregnancy.

AETIOLOGY Essential hypertension in >90–95% (cause unknown). Remainder are secondary to: *endocrine* (Cushing's, phaeochromocytoma, CAH), *renal* (renal artery stenosis, chronic renal disease), *vascular* (e.g. coarctation of aorta).

ASSOCIATIONS/RISK FACTORS Increasing age, ethnicity (Afro-Caribbean), obesity, smoking, diabetes, family history, pre-eclampsia.

EPIDEMIOLOGY Affects 1–5% of pregnancies.

HISTORY Largely asymptomatic.

EXAMINATION Blood pressure may be normal in first trimester due to ↓ systemic vascular resistance. Secondary causes include renal bruits, radiofemoral delay.

PATHOLOGY/PATHOGENESIS Chronic systemic inflammatory response increases susceptibility to pre-eclampsia. Placental pathology similar to pre-eclampsia (arterial occlusive changes, excess villous syncytial knots, infarction etc.) leads to hypoperfusion of the maternal space.

INVESTIGATIONS
Bloods: FBC, U&E, LFT, Urate.
Urinalysis: For proteinuria. If secondary causes are suspected: urinary catecholamines, renal artery USS and so on.
Fetus: Serial USS for fetal growth.

MANAGEMENT
Medication: Convert to non-teratogenic medications: methyldopa, nifedipine, labetalol (*note:* ACE inhibitors are teratogenic), aspirin 75 mg od (↓ risk of pre-eclampsia/IUGR).
Other: Monitor for pre-eclampsia, serial USS for fetal growth, uterine artery Dopplers at 24/40 (predicts pre-eclampsia).

COMPLICATIONS IUGR, superimposed pre-eclampsia (25%), placental abruption, prematurity.

PROGNOSIS Raised maternal and perinatal morbidity is related to superimposed pre-eclampsia.

Cord prolapse

DEFINITION Descent of the umbilical cord through the cervix past the presenting part in the presence of ruptured membranes: an *obstetric emergency*.

AETIOLOGY Potential space (e.g. unengaged presenting part) allows descent of the cord past the presenting part.

ASSOCIATIONS/RISK FACTORS Breech presentation, abnormal lie, multiple pregnancy (second twin), prematurity, low birthweight, unengaged presenting part, polyhydramnios, ARM.

EPIDEMIOLOGY Affects 0.1–0.6% of pregnancies.

HISTORY An abnormal FHR is detected, often after membrane rupture.

EXAMINATION Cord is felt or seen through the cervix below the presenting part.

PATHOLOGY/PATHOGENESIS Compression of the cord by the presenting part and arterial spasm prevents blood flow through the cord, causing asphyxia.

INVESTIGATIONS Unnecessary.

MANAGEMENT Place patient in Trendelenberg or knee–chest position. Manually elevate the presenting part (this may also be achieved through bladder filling). Emergency delivery is necessary, usually via Caesarean section. The neonatal team should be present at delivery.

COMPLICATIONS Hypoxic–ischaemic encephalopathy, fetal death.

PROGNOSIS Perinatal mortality rate is 91 per 1000, higher if it occurs outside hospital.

Diabetes in pregnancy

DEFINITION Pre-existing or new-onset diabetes in pregnancy.

AETIOLOGY
Pre-existing: Type 1 – failure of pancreas to produce insulin; type 2 – relative insulin deficiency associated with increased peripheral insulin resistance.
Gestational diabetes (GDM): Altered glucose tolerance in pregnancy.

ASSOCIATIONS/RISK FACTORS
GDM: ↑ maternal age, ethnicity (South Asian, Middle Eastern, Afro-Caribbean), obesity, smoking, PCOS, family history, previous macrosomic baby.

EPIDEMIOLOGY Prevalence is 2–5% but estimates vary. GDM accounts for 90% of diabetes in pregnancy.

HISTORY
Pre-existing: Usually known to mother.
GDM: Usually asymptomatic, detected on screening.

EXAMINATION
Abdomen: Fundal height (macrosomia/polyhydramnios).

PATHOLOGY/PATHOGENESIS
Type I: Autoimmune destruction of pancreatic islet cells.
Type II: Genetic component + influence of age and obesity on peripheral insulin resistance.
GDM: ↑ insulin resistance in pregnancy (↑ secretion of insulin antagonists, including HPL, glucagon and cortisol), altered carbohydrate metabolism, failure of normal pregnancy increase in insulin production.
Fetus: Hyperglycaemia in early pregnancy may affect development (congenital abnormalities); hyperglycaemia causes fetal hyperinsulinaemia and macrosomia.
Neonatal: Hypoglycaemia can occur (withdrawal of maternal glucose while fetal insulin levels remain high).

INVESTIGATIONS
Delivery: Aim for delivery after 38 completed weeks of pregnancy. Sliding scale in labour.
Pre-existing: Detailed anomaly scan, fetal cardiac scan, ophthalmic examination.
GDM: Screening (universal or selective) by GTT at 26–28/40.

MANAGEMENT
Pre-existing
Preconceptual: Optimisation of glucose control.
Medical: Optimise diet, consider converting oral hypoglycaemics to insulin. Likely to require increasing doses of insulin.
Pregnancy: Capillary blood glucose monitoring, monitor for pre-eclampsia, serial USS for fetal growth.
Delivery: Sliding scale in labour.
Postpartum: Return to pre-pregnancy doses of medications.

GDM
Medical: Diet control. Persistent hyperglycaemia may require insulin treatment.
Pregnancy/delivery: As for pre-existing.
Postpartum: Stop insulin after delivery, fasting blood glucose 6/52 postpartum.

COMPLICATIONS
Maternal: Progression of pre-existing nephropathy/neuropathy/retinopathy, miscarriage, pre-eclampsia, operative delivery.

Diabetes in pregnancy (continued)

Fetal/neonatal: Congenital abnormalities (pre-existing only), fetal death, polyhydramnios, polycythaemia, macrosomia (+ traumatic delivery), respiratory distress syndrome, neonatal hypoglycaemia, neonatal jaundice.

PROGNOSIS Dependent on adequacy of control.

GDM: 70% recurrence in future pregnancies, ↑ risk (40–60%) for type 2 diabetes.

Eclampsia

DEFINITION Grand mal seizures on a background of pre-eclampsia.

AETIOLOGY Unclear: see pathology/pathogenesis.

ASSOCIATIONS/RISK FACTORS Pre-existing pre-eclampsia.

EPIDEMIOLOGY UK incidence is 4.9 per 10 000 maternities, 44% postpartum, 18% intrapartum and 38% antenatal.

HISTORY Symptoms of impending eclampsia: headache, epigastric tenderness, visual disturbance, oedema, previous examination findings of hyperreflexia, clonus.

EXAMINATION Grand mal seizure.

PATHOLOGY/PATHOGENESIS Unclear. Mechanism related to cerebral vasospasm, hypertensive encephalopathy, tissue oedema, ischaemia and haemorrhage have been proposed.

INVESTIGATIONS
Bloods: (As for pre-eclampsia) FBC, clotting, U&E, urate, LFT, G&S, consider ABG.
Urine: ? proteinuria.
Imaging (post-seizure): CT head, CXR if chest signs.

MANAGEMENT
Airway and breathing: Apply oxygen, maintain patency, ventilation if appropriate.
Circulation: Manage on left tilt, ensure large-bore IV access, evaluate pulse and blood pressure.
Drugs: IV magnesium sulphate: 4 g loading dose followed by 1 g/h (monitor urine output, respiratory rate, patellar reflexes).
Recurrent seizures: Consider – further bolus magnesium sulphate, thiopentone, diazepam, IPPV and muscle relaxation.
Post-seizure: Assess chest, control blood pressure (consider IV labetalol/hydralazine), strict fluid management, (85 mL/h input, urine output >25 mL/h), may require CVP monitoring, deliver baby (only when mother stabilised), consider ITU.

COMPLICATIONS Cardiac arrest, death, permanent CNS damage (e.g. cortical blindness), CVA (1–2%), DIC, renal failure, ARDS.

PROGNOSIS Maternal mortality rate 1.8%; significant morbidity in 35%.

Epilepsy in pregnancy

DEFINITION A continuing tendency to have seizures.

AETIOLOGY Usually idiopathic.

ASSOCIATIONS/RISK FACTORS Family history, intracranial mass, previous intracranial surgery, head injury, cerebrovascular disease, CNS infections.

EPIDEMIOLOGY Affects 0.5% women of childbearing age.

HISTORY Known personal history of epilepsy.

EXAMINATION Often unremarkable.

PATHOLOGY/PATHOGENESIS
Seizure: Paroxysmal discharge of cerebral neurones results in convulsions.
Seizure types: Primary generalised, partial (focal) or complex partial, temporal lobe.
Altered seizure frequency in pregnancy: Related to ↑ renal and hepatic drug clearance,
↑ volume of distribution, ↓ absorption (e.g. during labour, nausea and vomiting),
compliance issues (fear of congenital abnormalities).

INVESTIGATIONS
Bloods: (Effects of anticonvulsants) FBC (↑MCV), serum folate, serum anticonvulsant levels,
LFT.
Fetus: Detailed fetal anomaly scan ± fetal echo.

MANAGEMENT
Preconceptual: Maximise control on least teratogenic monotherapy if possible, folic acid
5 mg od.
Medication: Remains the same (benefits outweigh risks of changing) if well controlled with
phenytoin, carbamazepine, lamotrigine, valproate, phenobaritone or levetiracetam (may
require ↑ doses and may need to monitor drug levels). If diagnosed in pregnancy,
lamotrigine and carbamazepine are drugs of choice. Vitamin K from 36/40 if
enzyme-inducing drugs taken.
Delivery: Continue medications, may require diazepam/lorazepam if seizures during labour.
Postnatal: IM neonatal vitamin K. Gradually reduce doses of any medications increased in
pregnancy to baseline.

COMPLICATIONS
Maternal: Change in seizure frequency, causes around 5 maternal deaths a year in UK.
Fetal: Teratogenicity related to antiepileptic drugs – congenital abnormalities (orofacial,
neural tube, congenital heart), ↑ risk childhood epilepsy, haemorrhagic disease of the
newborn (if enzyme-inducing drugs taken).

PROGNOSIS Poorly controlled/multiple seizure types more likely to deteriorate in
pregnancy. Long-term seizure-free patients unlikely to experience an increase in seizures.
Highest risk is peri-partum.

Fetal distress in labour

DEFINITION Fetal hypoxia in labour, ± acidosis. Diagnosis is by intermittent auscultation, continuous CTG or FBS.

AETIOLOGY Insufficient oxygen transfer from mother to fetus results in an asphyxial insult.

ASSOCIATIONS/RISK FACTORS Hypertonic uterus, placental insufficiency, intrauterine infection, cord prolapse, placental abruption, IUGR, oligohydramnios, post-dates pregnancy, hypertensive disease.

EPIDEMIOLOGY UK incidence: 2–10% (note: diagnosis of fetal distress necessitates delivery).

HISTORY Detected via monitoring, ?features of underlying condition (e.g. hypertension, abruption).

EXAMINATION
General: Assess maternal pulse (maternal tachycardia can cause fetal tachycardia), BP (maternal hypovolaemia), temperature (signs of infection/chorioamnionitis).
Abdomen: Check for hypertonic/irritable uterus (hyperstimulation, abruption), clinical assessment of fetal growth/liquor (IUGR, oligohydramnios).
Vaginal: Assess cervical dilatation, colour of liquor, bleeding, check for cord prolapse.

PATHOLOGY/PATHOGENESIS Impairment of transfer of O_2 and CO_2 between mother and fetus (e.g. due to placental insufficiency/pathology, fetal conditions resulting in reduced oxygen-carrying capacity such as anaemia, infection) leads to hypoxia. Excess CO_2 is converted to carbonic acid, causing a respiratory acidosis and leading to a fall in pH. Buffering system exists to attempt to maintain pH. Can recover if oxygenation re-established. If insult is prolonged, lactate accumulates leading to metabolic acidosis – pH falls and base excess rises.

INVESTIGATIONS
Bloods: FBC, G&S (preparation for delivery).
CTG
FBS: pH >7.25 is reassuring unless CTG continues to deteriorate, <7.25 repeat at 30 mins (note: <7.2 requires delivery).

MANAGEMENT
General: Left tilt, IV access, stop oxytocin infusion if in progress.
Fetal bradycardia >6 minutes: Necessitates emergency delivery.
Persistent CTG abnormalities: (See Cardiotocography appendix) may require FBS.
Delivery: If fully dilated, <1/5 palpable abdominally and vertex at or below spines, consider instrumental delivery. Otherwise deliver by Caesarean section.

COMPLICATIONS
Maternal: Complications of operative delivery.
Fetal: Hypoxic ischaemic encephalopathy, death.

PROGNOSIS Depends on underlying cause and timeliness of intervention.

Group B streptococcal infection

DEFINITION Group B *Streptococcus* (GBS) is the most common cause of early-onset (<7 days) infection in neonates.

AETIOLOGY Commensal bacterium of the vagina and rectum, carried by 25% of women. Of the babies who come into contact with GBS during labour the majority will not be affected. Some will become colonised. A minority become seriously ill, often within the first 12 hours after delivery.

ASSOCIATIONS/RISK FACTORS Positive HVS/LVS/rectal swab/MSU, previously affected baby, pyrexia in labour, prolonged rupture of membranes, PTL.

EPIDEMIOLOGY Most frequent cause of early-onset neonatal infection. Incidence is 0.5 per 1000 births in UK.

HISTORY Often asymptomatic. Detected on MSU, HVS or LVS. ?Prolonged rupture of membranes. ?PTL.

EXAMINATION Usually unremarkable.

PATHOLOGY/PATHOGENESIS Gram-positive *Streptococcus* characterised by the presence of Group B Lancefield antigen. Also known as *Streptococcus agalactiae*.

INVESTIGATIONS

Microbiology: HVS, LVS, rectal swab for MC&S. There is no national screening programme for GBS in the UK (no clear evidence of benefit, and concerns about antibiotic resistance/anaphylaxis).

MANAGEMENT IV antibiotics in labour (benzylpenicillin, clindamycin if penicllin-allergic). If detected antenatally on MSU, treat with antibiotics.

COMPLICATIONS

Neonatal: Septicaemia, pneumonia, meningitis, death.

PROGNOSIS Treatment is 80% effective in preventing early-onset GBS infection. Mortality is 10% in early-onset neonatal infection.

HIV in pregnancy

DEFINITION Human immunodeficiency virus – a retrovirus that attacks T lymphocytes.

AETIOLOGY HIV is present in vaginal fluid, semen, blood and breast milk of infected patients. Transmission: sexual contact, blood-borne, vertical.

ASSOCIATIONS/RISK FACTORS Increased risk of vertical transmission with ↑ viral load, ↓ CD4 count, prolonged rupture of membranes (>4 hours), breastfeeding.

EPIDEMIOLOGY Increasingly common due to increased life expectancy in individuals with HIV infection. Prevalence 0.38% in London, 0.06% in rest of UK.

HISTORY May be asymptomatic until progression to AIDS (average 8–10 years). ?Febrile seroconversion illness.

EXAMINATION No clinical features in HIV. May present with opportunistic infection, or rarely AIDS-defining illness (e.g. *Pneumocystis carinii* pneumonia (PCP), Kaposi's sarcoma, oesophageal candidiasis).

PATHOLOGY/PATHOGENESIS In women who do not breastfeed, over 80% vertical transmission occurs late in the third trimester (>36 weeks) and at delivery. Less than 2% occurs in the first two trimesters.

INVESTIGATIONS
Bloods: Routine HIV testing at antenatal booking. Regular viral load and CD4 count.
Monitoring for drug toxicity: FBC, U&E, LFT, lactate and blood glucose.

MANAGEMENT
Antenatal: HAART (a combination of at least three antiretrovirals) if CD4 count >350 × 10^6/L. Aim to suppress viral load to undetectable levels (<50 copies/mL). If CD4 count and viral load acceptable, can start antiretrovirals from 28 to 32 weeks.
Intrapartum: If viral load detectable or non-compliant with HAART, advise Caesarean section. IV zidovudine infusion given from 4 h prior to delivery until cord is clamped.
Viral load undetectable: Consider vaginal delivery, avoid FBS/FSE or rupture of membranes for >4 h.
Neonatal: Antiretrovirals for 4–6 weeks, PCR testing at birth, 3 weeks, 6 weeks and 6 months, HIV antibody test at 18 months. Avoid breastfeeding.

COMPLICATIONS Side-effects of HAART – pre-eclampsia, obstetric cholestasis and other liver dysfunction, lactic acidosis, glucose intolerance, GDM.

PROGNOSIS No evidence to suggest that pregnancy accelerates progression to AIDS. Appropriate measures as above reduce transmission rate from 28% to <2%.

Infections in pregnancy – *chicken pox*

DEFINITION Primary infection caused by the varicella zoster virus.

AETIOLOGY Transmission by physical contact, aerosol route, vertical.

ASSOCIATIONS/RISK FACTORS No prior immunity, immigrant population from tropical or subtropical areas (*note:* can be transmitted via patients with shingles).

EPIDEMIOLOGY Complicates 3 per 1000 pregnancies, 90% immunity in women in the UK.

HISTORY Fever, malaise, pruritic rash (becomes vesicular then crusts over).

EXAMINATION Vesicular rash.

PATHOLOGY/PATHOGENESIS DNA virus (herpes family), highly infectious.
Spread: Aerosol route, direct contact with vesicular fluid, indirectly via fomites.
Incubation period: 1–3 weeks, infectious from 48 hours prior to the rash forming until vesicles crust over.
Dormant period: Following primary infection the virus lies dormant in sensory nerve root ganglia and may reactivate as shingles.

INVESTIGATIONS
Bloods: Varicella zoster IgM (active infection) or IgG (immunity).
USS: Fetal anomaly scan (fetal varicella syndrome).

MANAGEMENT
Non-immune mother: Give VZIG.
Established chicken pox: Aciclovir (800 mg 5 × daily for 7 days), if within 24 h of onset of rash (caution prior to 20 weeks).
Maternal infection near term: Avoid elective delivery for 5–7 days after rash appears (allows placental transfer of maternal antibodies).
Neonate: Requires VZIG if delivered within 7 days before or after onset of maternal rash.

COMPLICATIONS
Maternal: Pneumonia (10%), hepatitis, encephalitis, death (rare).
Fetal: Fetal varicella syndrome (if maternal infection before 28/40): skin scarring, eye defects, limb deformities, neurological abnormalities.
Neonatal: Varicella infection of the newborn (if maternal infection 1–4 weeks prior to delivery to 1 week postpartum).

PROGNOSIS After exposure, VZIG reduces risk of maternal infection to 50% in the non-immune. No increased risk of miscarriage.

Infections in pregnancy – *cytomegalovirus*

DEFINITION Common viral infection, associated with a severe congenital syndrome in the fetus.

AETIOLOGY

Transmission: Sexual contact, blood-borne, contact with infected bodily fluids (saliva or urine), vertical.

ASSOCIATIONS/RISK FACTORS Higher socioeconomic class (less likely to have immunity through childhood infection), immunosuppression (e.g. HIV).

EPIDEMIOLOGY There is 50% immunity in pregnant women. 1% of seronegative pregnant women will contract CMV antenatally.

HISTORY Often asymptomatic, ?fever, malaise, fatigue.

EXAMINATION Often no clinical signs, ?lymphadenopathy.

PATHOLOGY/PATHOGENESIS DNA virus (herpes family). Following primary infection can remain dormant and then reactivate (e.g. in immunosuppression). Incubation period 1–2 months.

INVESTIGATIONS

Bloods: CMV IgM (current infection)/IgG (immunity).
USS: Fetal anomaly scan.
Other: Amniocentesis for CMV PCR (6–9 weeks after primary infection).

MANAGEMENT No treatment to prevent transmission to fetus. May offer termination of pregnancy if evidence of CNS damage. Neonatal gancyclovir can attenuate audiological complications.

COMPLICATIONS Increased risk of miscarriage and stillbirth, congenital CMV (IUGR, microcephaly, intracerebral calcification, blindness, sensori-neural deafness, hepatosplenomegaly, skin rash, pneumonitis, mental retardation).

PROGNOSIS Rate of transmission to the fetus is 40%. Of these, 10% will develop the congenital syndrome. Ninety percent of babies who are symptomatic at birth will have later neuro-developmental problems.

Infections in pregnancy – *hepatitis B*

DEFINITION Infection caused by the hepatitis B virus.

AETIOLOGY Transmission by sexual contact, blood-borne, vertical.

ASSOCIATIONS/RISK FACTORS Multiple sexual partners, unprotected sexual intercourse, intravenous drug use, ↑ prevalence in South-East Asian immigrant population.

EPIDEMIOLOGY Affects 1 per 100 000 pregnancies.

HISTORY Fever, myalgia, nausea, vomiting, jaundice, abdominal pain (*note:* asymptomatic in 70%).

EXAMINATION Jaundice, hepatomegaly, right upper quadrant tenderness.

PATHOLOGY/PATHOGENESIS Double-stranded DNA virus (Hepadanavirus family) replicates in the liver and causes hepatic dysfunction. Incubation period 2–6 months.

INVESTIGATIONS
Bloods: HBsAg (infection), core antibody (anti-HBc IgM – acute infection), hepatitis B e-markers (HBeAg – high infectivity), LFTs.

MANAGEMENT
Delivery: Caesarean section is *not* indicated, avoid FBS/FSE.
Postnatal: Mothers *can* breastfeed.
Neonatal vaccination: (If mother is HBsAg positive) at birth, 1 month, 2 months and booster at 1 year.
Neonatal HBIG: (Within 48 h of delivery) appropriate if birthweight <1500 g, if acute infection occurred in pregnancy, if mother is HBeAg positive or HBeAg negative + anti-HBe negative, or if e-markers are unknown.

COMPLICATIONS
Maternal: 10% develop chronic disease (chronic hepatitis, cirrhosis), ↑ risk of hepatocellular carcinoma, 1% develop fulminating hepatitis.
Neonates: 90% of babies infected with hepatitis B develop chronic hepatitis.

PROGNOSIS With appropriate treatment, vertical transmission rate is 10%.

Infections in pregnancy – *herpes simplex*

DEFINITION Infection caused by the herpes simplex virus (HSV).

AETIOLOGY Transmission by physical contact, sexual contact, vertical.

ASSOCIATIONS/RISK FACTORS Unprotected sexual intercourse, immunosuppression (e.g. HIV), other STIs.

EPIDEMIOLOGY Herpes simplex infects 2% of pregnant women.

HISTORY Burning sensation, pain, pruritis, dysuria (*note:* may be asymptomatic).

EXAMINATION Clusters of vesicles with surrounding erythema, can progress to ulcerated lesions which crust over, ?associated lymphadenopathy.

PATHOLOGY/PATHOGENESIS DNA virus (herpes family) of two types – 1: oral, 2: genital.

Dormant period: Following primary infection, HSV remains dormant in nerve ganglia and can be reactivated to form recurrent lesions.

Spread to neonate: Mainly direct contact with infected maternal secretions (but transplacental transmission possible), risk of neonatal transmission at vaginal delivery – 41% with primary lesions, 2% with recurrent lesions.

INVESTIGATIONS Usually diagnosed clinically.

Microbiology: Swabs for viral culture/PCR, STI screen.

Bloods: HSV antibody (primary infection in third trimester).

MANAGEMENT

Antenatal: Aciclovir (200 mg 5 × daily for 5 days) in primary infection.

Delivery with primary HSV: If within 6 weeks of likely delivery, advise Caesarean section. If opts for vaginal delivery, give IV aciclovir intrapartum, avoid prolonged ruptured membranes/FSE/FBS.

Delivery with recurrent HSV: Does not necessitate Caesarean section. Women may opt for Caesarean if lesions detected at onset of labour – can offer daily aciclovir from 36/40 to reduce likelihood of lesions.

COMPLICATIONS

Maternal: Disseminated herpes (encephalitis, hepatitis, disseminated skin lesions) rare but more common in pregnancy.

Neonatal: 1 per 60 000 live births – can affect skin/eyes/mouth, CNS or multiple organs.

PROGNOSIS Neonatal mortality from 2% (local disease) to 50% (disseminated disease).

Infections in pregnancy – *listeriosis*

DEFINITION Infection caused by the bacterium *Listeria monocytogenes*.

AETIOLOGY Found in soil, decayed matter and animals. Transmission by faeco-oral route (soft cheese, paté, unpasteurised dairy products, unwashed salads), vertical (transplacentally or during delivery).

ASSOCIATIONS/RISK FACTORS Increased risk of infection in pregnancy and immunosuppression.

EPIDEMIOLOGY Rare: 1 per 20 000 pregnancies in UK.

HISTORY Diarrhoea, vomiting, malaise, fever, sore throat, myalgia (*note*: often asymptomatic).

EXAMINATION No specific signs.

PATHOLOGY/PATHOGENESIS Gram-positive bacillus, transmission as noted above.

INVESTIGATIONS
Microbiology: Blood culture, amniotic fluid culture, placental culture (*note*: serological testing is not reliable).

MANAGEMENT IV antibiotics (penicillin and aminoglycoside, e.g. gentamicin).

COMPLICATIONS
General: Septicaemia, pneumonia, meningitis.
Pregnancy: Miscarriage, chorioamnionitis, PTL, fetal death.

PROGNOSIS Good prognosis if treated; poor prognosis with septicaemia (mortality 50%), meningitis (70%) or if neonatal infection occurs (80%).

Infections in pregnancy – *parvovirus B19*

DEFINITION Erythema infectiosum (Fifth disease) caused by parvovirus B19.

AETIOLOGY Transmission by aerosol route, also blood-borne.

ASSOCIATIONS/RISK FACTORS Most commonly affects children but also affects susceptible adults.

EPIDEMIOLOGY Common infection, with 60% immunity in adults by age 20 years. Affects 1 per 400 pregnancies.

HISTORY Rash, malaise, fever, arthropathy (*note:* 25% of cases are asymptomatic).

EXAMINATION Rash – commonly 'slapped cheek' appearance (erythema infectiosum). May have purpura, erythema multiforme.

PATHOLOGY/PATHOGENESIS Small single-stranded DNA virus, incubation period 13–20 days. Infective from 10 days prior to onset of rash until appearance of rash. Risk period of transmission to fetus is between 4/40 and 20/40. No intrauterine transmission under 4/40. Low risk of fetal hydrops after 20/40.

INVESTIGATIONS
Bloods: Parvovirus serology IgM (active infection), IgG (immunity), rubella serology (similar presentation).
USS: Fetal anomaly scan 4 weeks after onset of illness, and then at 1–2 weekly intervals until 30/40.

MANAGEMENT
Maternal: Symptomatic treatment (mild, self-limiting illness).
Fetus: Intrauterine blood transfusion (if fetal hydrops).

COMPLICATIONS
Maternal: Aplastic anaemia, arthritis, myocarditis, nephritis.
Fetus: Miscarriage (15%), fetal hydrops (3%).

PROGNOSIS Untreated fetal hydrops has 50% mortality (reduced to 18% by intrauterine blood transfusion). Does not cause congenital abnormalities.

Infections in pregnancy – *rubella*

DEFINITION Infection caused by the rubella virus.

AETIOLOGY Transmission by aerosol route, vertical (transplacental).

ASSOCIATIONS/RISK FACTORS Non-immunity (↑ rates in ethnic minorities).

EPIDEMIOLOGY Rare: 97% of women are vaccinated or immune in the UK.

HISTORY Fever, malaise, coryzal symptoms, arthralgia, rash.

EXAMINATION Lymphadenopathy, maculopapular rash (usually starting behind the ears, spreading to head and neck, then to the rest of the body).

PATHOLOGY/PATHOGENESIS RNA virus (Togaviridae family) with incubation period 6–21 days, infectious from 1 week prior to 5 days after onset of rash.

INVESTIGATIONS
Bloods: Rubella serology IgM (active infection), IgG (immunity).
USS: Fetal anomaly.

MANAGEMENT Symptomatic treatment of mother. May offer TOP if confirmed infection in first trimester.

COMPLICATIONS
Maternal: Miscarriage, pneumonia, arthropathy, encephalitis, ITP.
Fetal: Death, congenital rubella syndrome (deafness, VSD, PDA, cataracts, CNS defects, IUGR, hepatosplenomegaly, thrombocytopenia, rash).

PROGNOSIS Highest risk is congenital rubella syndrome with infection in first trimester (90%), 5–10% risk between 14 and 16/40, low risk after 20/40. Rubella and congenital rubella syndrome very rare owing to routine childhood vaccination since 1988 (MMR).

Infections in pregnancy – *toxoplasmosis*

DEFINITION Infection caused by the protozoon *Toxoplasma gondii*.

AETIOLOGY Transmission by faeco-oral route (found in infected meat and cat faeces).

ASSOCIATIONS/RISK FACTORS Household cats, ↑ incidence in rural areas, ↑ incidence in France.

EPIDEMIOLOGY Affects 1 per 2000 pregnancies.

HISTORY Fever, malaise, arthralgia (*note:* often asymptomatic).

EXAMINATION No specific clinical signs, ?fever/lymphadenopathy.

PATHOLOGY/PATHOGENESIS Parasite excreted in cat faeces, with incubation period 5–23 days. ↑ risk of vertical transmission with increasing gestational age (5% in the first trimester, 80% in the third trimester). However risk of congenital toxoplasmosis *reduces* with increasing gestational age (60–80% in the first trimester, 5% in the third trimester).

INVESTIGATIONS
Bloods: Toxoplasma IgM (active infection), IgG (immunity).
USS: Fetal anomaly scan.
Other: Amniocentesis (to detect fetal infection).

MANAGEMENT
Antibiotics: Spiramycin (↓ risk of vertical transmission).
Termination: May offer termination of pregnancy with USS evidence of fetal infection.

COMPLICATIONS Miscarriage, PTL, fetal death, congenital toxoplasmosis (hydrocephalus, retinochoroiditis, intracranial calcification, IUGR, hepatosplenomegaly, thrombocytopenia, rash).

PROGNOSIS Dependent on the severity of congenital toxoplasmosis.

Intrauterine death

DEFINITION Death of a fetus after 24/40.

AETIOLOGY

Maternal: Prolonged pregnancy, diabetes, pre-eclampsia, hypertension, obstetric cholestasis, SLE, antiphospholipid syndrome, thrombophilias, infections, Rhesus isoimmunisation, haemoglobinopathies, uterine rupture, maternal trauma, maternal death.

Fetal: Congenital abnormalities, genetic abnormalities, IUGR, infections (parvovirus, listeria, TORCH), hydrops fetalis, multiple gestation.

Placental: Placental insufficiency, abruption, vasa praevia.

Intrapartum factors: Birth asphyxia, shoulder dystocia, cord accident.

Other: Idiopathic.

ASSOCIATIONS/RISK FACTORS As for aetiology; also associated with ↑ maternal age, smoking, recreational drug use, previous intrauterine death.

EPIDEMIOLOGY Affects 5 per 1000 pregnancies.

HISTORY Reduced or absent fetal movements, symptoms of underlying conditions.

EXAMINATION

Abdomen: Absent FH, may have↓ fundal height, features of underlying conditions.

PATHOLOGY/PATHOGENESIS Dependent on the cause.

INVESTIGATIONS

USS: Confirm absent fetal heart movements (two accredited operators).

Bloods: FBC, U&E, LFT, CRP, HbA1c, clotting, thrombophilia screen, TORCH screen, parvovirus serology, Kleihauer (feto-maternal haemorrhage).

Other: Placental histology, fetal karyotype, post mortem.

MANAGEMENT Offer induction of labour.

Post-delivery: Offer bromocriptine or cabergoline to suppress lactation, arrange bereavement counselling, discuss consent for post mortem, follow-up with results.

COMPLICATIONS DIC, postnatal depression.

PROGNOSIS Unlikely to recur if no cause found, but manage subsequent pregnancies as 'high risk'.

Intrauterine growth restriction

DEFINITION Slowing of fetal growth such that it fails to reach its growth potential.

AETIOLOGY

Maternal: Hypertension, pre-eclampsia, diabetes, drug/alcohol abuse, smoking, renal disease, thrombophilia, ↑maternal age.

Fetal: Chromosomal abnormalities, infection (e.g. CMV, rubella), multiple pregnancy.

Other: Placental insufficiency.

ASSOCIATIONS/RISK FACTORS As for aetiology; previous IUGR.

EPIDEMIOLOGY Affects 3–5% of pregnancies.

HISTORY History of any aetiological factors noted above; enquire about fetal movements.

EXAMINATION

Abdomen: ↓fundal height.

PATHOLOGY/PATHOGENESIS

Symmetrical IUGR: Head and body are proportionally small, normally early onset, seen in chromosomal abnormalities.

Asymmetrical IUGR: Typically later onset, abdominal circumference disproportionately smaller than the head, seen with placental insufficiency.

INVESTIGATIONS

USS: Anomaly scan, growth (abdominal and head circumference), liquor volume (?oligohydramnios), umbilical artery Doppler (abnormal if end-diastolic flow absent or reversed), middle cerebral artery Doppler (may show redistribution of blood to brain).

CTG: Fetal wellbeing.

MANAGEMENT

Normal Doppler results: Aim delivery >37/40 unless abnormalities arise, with regular fetal monitoring.

Abnormal Doppler results: Steroids if pre-term, consider delivery, paediatrician at delivery, continuous CTG intrapartum.

COMPLICATIONS Stillbirth, PTL, intrapartum fetal distress, birth asphyxia, meconium aspiration, postnatal hypoglycaemia, neurodevelopmental delay, ↑ risk type 2 diabetes and hypertension in adult life.

PROGNOSIS Increased perinatal morbidity and mortality, increased neurodevelopmental delay if onset <26/40.

Malposition

DEFINITION Abnormal position of fetal vertex in relation to the maternal pelvis.

AETIOLOGY Fetal head normally engages in the OT position, rotating to the OA position with simultaneous flexion. Malpositions in labour include OP, OT and deflexion of the head.

ASSOCIATIONS/RISK FACTORS Cephalopelvic disproportion (e.g. android pelvis), epidural, inadequate uterine contractions.

EPIDEMIOLOGY Ten percent of labours start OP, most correct during labour.

HISTORY ? Prolonged labour.

EXAMINATION
Abdomen: OP suspected if the lower abdomen appears flattened.
Vaginal: Determine position through palpation of fetal fontanelles, assess for caput/ moulding.

PATHOLOGY/PATHOGENESIS NA.

INVESTIGATIONS
CTG: For fetal wellbeing, frequency of contractions.
Bloods: FBC, G&S (preparation for delivery).

MANAGEMENT
Labour: Hydrate, augment with oxytocin infusion, offer epidural ($\uparrow$ likelihood obstetric intervention, $\downarrow$ urge to push prior to full dilatation if OP).
Delivery: (If failure to progress) if fully dilated, <1/5 palpable abdominally and vertex at or below spines – vaginal delivery with manual rotation/Kielland's forceps/rotational ventouse delivery. Otherwise offer Caesarean section.

COMPLICATIONS
Maternal: Exhaustion, risks obstetric intervention.
Fetal: Fetal distress, complications of instrumental delivery.

PROGNOSIS Good; 75% of OP positions spontaneously rotate to OA.

Malpresentation

DEFINITION Any presentation where the presenting part is not the fetal vertex.

AETIOLOGY Associated with fetal/maternal factors that affect rotation.

ASSOCIATIONS/RISK FACTORS
Maternal: Placental site abnormalities, uterine abnormalities, obstructed lower segment (fibroids, pelvic abnormalities) grand multiparity (uterine laxity).
Fetal: Multiple gestation, prematurity, fetal malformation, polyhydramnios, macrosomia.

EPIDEMIOLOGY Prevalence at term: breech 3–4%, transverse lie 0.3%, face 0.002%, brow 0.001%, compound 0.1%.

HISTORY Asymptomatic, detected on examination.

EXAMINATION
Breech
Abdomen: Palpable head at fundus, soft breech in pelvis.
Vaginal: Soft presenting part, ischial tuberosities, anus or genitalia may be felt.
Footling breech: Foot felt/seen through the cervix.

Transverse lie
Abdomen: No presenting part felt in pelvis, uterus appears wide, fundal height may be low.
Vaginal: No presenting part felt in pelvis.

Face
Vaginal: Facial landmarks felt.

Brow
Vaginal: Supraorbital ridges ± base of nose felt.

PATHOLOGY/PATHOGENESIS NA.

INVESTIGATIONS
Breech or transverse: USS to confirm lie.

MANAGEMENT
Breech
ECV may be attempted after 37 weeks.

Persistent breech: Recommend Caesarean section (↑ fetal/neonatal morbidity with vaginal delivery).

Transverse lie
Requires delivery by Caesarean section, ECV occasionally attempted.

Brow
If persistent or second stage, deliver by Caesarean section.

Face
Mentoposterior position: Deliver by Caesarean section.
Mentoanterior: May attempt vaginal delivery.

Compound
Commonly this is fetal arm alongside fetal head – manage expectantly.

COMPLICATIONS
Maternal: Morbidity resulting from operative delivery, prolonged/obstructed labour, uterine rupture (especially transverse), PPH, ↑ perineal injury (mentoanterior face presentation).

Malpresentation (continued)

Fetal: ↑ perinatal mortality/morbidity (difficult delivery, prematurity, congenital abnormalities), cord prolapse (asphyxia).

PROGNOSIS Dependent on aetiology, presentation and timeliness of appropriate management.

Multiple pregnancy

DEFINITION Pregnancy involving more than one fetus.

AETIOLOGY

Monozygous: Division of fertilised egg – DCDA: splitting 3 days, 2 chorions, 2 amnions; MCDA: splitting 4–7 days, single placenta, one chorion, 2 amnions; MCMA: splitting 8–12 days, single placenta, one amnion, one chorion.

Dizygous: Fertilisation of >1 ovum by different sperm – DCDA: separate placentae, amnions and chorions.

ASSOCIATIONS/RISK FACTORS Previous history, family history, ovulation, African race, ↑ maternal age.

EPIDEMIOLOGY Incidence of twins, 11%; incidence of triplets, 1 per 8100.

HISTORY

First trimester: Incidental finding on ultrasound, hyperemesis (increased β-HCG).
Later in pregnancy: Large-for-dates, multiple fetal parts on abdominal examination.

EXAMINATION

Abdomen: ↑fundal height, multiple fetal parts, >1 FH.

PATHOLOGY/PATHOGENESIS NA.

INVESTIGATIONS Confirmation by USS: establishment of chorionicity (almost 100% accurate in first trimester only), nuchal translucency (*note:* serum screening unreliable).

MANAGEMENT

Antenatal: Serial USS for fetal growths (dichorionic: 4-weekly from 24/40; monochorionic: 2-weekly scans from 18 weeks), monitor FBC (↑ anaemia), monitor BP (↑ eclampsia), GTT (↑ diabetes).

Vaginal delivery: May be attempted if first twin cephalic (need continuous monitoring and active management in third stage).

Caesarean section: Recommended for delayed delivery of second twin, fetal distress of either twin, malpresentation of second twin after delivery of first (ECV or internal version may be attempted prior), non-vertex presentation of first twin, monoamniotic twins, higher order births.

COMPLICATIONS

Maternal: Miscarriage, hyperemesis, pre-eclampsia, anaemia (↑ plasma volume and fetal iron requirements), PPH, APH, diabetes (↑ steroid load), operative delivery, postnatal depression.

Fetal: Prematurity, polyhydramnios, congenital malformations, IUGR, fetal death, discordant growth.

Monochorionic twins: Twin–twin transfusion syndrome (placental anastomoses produce haemodynamic imbalance resulting in polyhydramnios and hydrops in one twin and oligohydramnios and IUGR in the other).

Intrapartum: Cord prolapse, twin interlocking, ↑ perinatal morbidity of second twin (vaginal delivery).

PROGNOSIS Dependent on complications; twin fetal mortality rate 4 times higher than singletons.

Obstetric cholestasis

DEFINITION Pruritis in pregnancy, which resolves on delivery, associated with abnormal liver function in the absence of any other identifiable pathology.

AETIOLOGY Complex, likely genetic and hormonal factors.

ASSOCIATIONS/RISK FACTORS Previous history, family history, ethnicity (South Asian, Chilean, Bolivian), multiple pregnancy.

EPIDEMIOLOGY UK prevalence: 0.7% of pregnancies.

HISTORY Normally occurs in the second half of pregnancy. Generalised pruritis in the absence of rash (often worse at night, may be more intense over the palms and soles), rarely associated with dark urine and steatorrhoea.

EXAMINATION Often entirely normal but excoriations may be present.

PATHOLOGY/PATHOGENESIS Increased susceptibility to cholestatic effect of oestrogens, ?related to impaired sulfation, may also be related to a defect in membrane phospholipid which may be inheritable.

INVESTIGATIONS

Bloods: LFT ($\uparrow$ transaminases/GGT, occasionally mild hyperbilirubinaemia, may be preceded by symptoms therefore consider fortnightly repeat if normal), bile acids (raised), clotting (may be abnormal due to $\downarrow$ vitamin K absorption).

Diagnosis of exclusion, therefore need: PET screen (FBC, U&E, LFT, clotting), liver USS, hepatitis serology (A, B, C and E), EBV and CMV serology, liver autoantibodies (AMA, ASMA).

MANAGEMENT

Monitoring: Weekly LFT and clotting, serial USS for fetal + intermittent CTG monitoring (limited in prediction of fetal compromise).

Medications: Chlorpheniramine (control pruritis), ursodeoxycholic acid ($\downarrow$ serum bile acids and pruritis, no effect on fetal compromise), vitamin K ($\downarrow$ fetal/maternal haemorrhage), dexamethasone (if no response to UCDA).

Delivery: Induce at 37/40 owing to increased risk of fetal death.

Postpartum: Ensure resolution of abnormal LFTs after 10/7 postpartum.

COMPLICATIONS

Maternal: PPH ($\downarrow$ vitamin K).

Fetal: Death, intracranial haemorrhage ($\downarrow$ vitamin K), fetal distress, preterm delivery.

PROGNOSIS Complete recovery is made postnatally, but 90% recurrence in future pregnancies. Risk of fetal death is 2–3%.

Oligohydramnios

DEFINITION Decreased volume of amniotic fluid, below fifth centile, or deepest pool less than 2 cm.

AETIOLOGY Rupture of membranes, placental insufficiency, fetal urinary tract pathology/ malformations.

ASSOCIATIONS/RISK FACTORS Chromosomal abnormalities, post-term pregnancies, IUGR, pre-eclampsia, medication (ACE inhibitors, indomethacin), multiple pregnancy (e.g. TTTS).

EPIDEMIOLOGY Affects 4% of pregnancies.

HISTORY History of fluid leak PV with rupture of membranes (*note:* commonly asymptomatic).

EXAMINATION
Abdomen: ↓ fundal height, fetal parts easily palpable.
Speculum: Assess for ruptured membranes if clinically appropriate.

PATHOLOGY/PATHOGENESIS Reduced amniotic fluid volume by loss of fluid or reduced fetal urine output (↓ placental function or fetal urinary tract pathology).

INVESTIGATIONS
USS: Diagnosis + assessment of liquor volume, fetal growth, umbilical artery Dopplers, exclude fetal anomalies.
CTG: Fetal wellbeing.

MANAGEMENT
If PROM/PPROM: See relevant sections.
Term: Delivery is appropriate (IOL if no contraindications).
Pre-term: Monitor with serial USS for growth, liquor volume and Dopplers, regular CTGs, deliver if further abnormalities arise (*note:* amnioinfusion has a very limited role in modern obstetrics).

COMPLICATIONS
Labour: ↑ incidence CTG abnormalities, meconium liquor, emergency Caesarean section.
Neonate: pulmonary hypoplasia, limb deformities.

PROGNOSIS Dependent on gestation at time of presentation: increased perinatal mortality rates with early-onset oligohydramnios.

Placental abruption

DEFINITION Separation of the placenta from the uterine wall prior to delivery.

AETIOLOGY Often idiopathic, may occur secondary to raised pressure on maternal side of placenta (e.g. hypertension) or mechanical trauma.

ASSOCIATIONS/RISK FACTORS Hypertensive disorders, previous history of abruption, PPROM, abdominal trauma, smoking, cocaine usage, polyhydramnios.

EPIDEMIOLOGY Affects 1–2% of pregnancies.

HISTORY Constant abdominal pain, PV bleed (if revealed).

EXAMINATION
General: ?shocked.
Abdomen: Hypertonic 'woody', tender uterus.
Speculum: Assess bleeding.
Vaginal: (Ensure not known placenta praevia) cervical dilatation (consider ARM if term and no fetal distress).
CTG: Fetal wellbeing.

PATHOLOGY/PATHOGENESIS As the placenta separates, retroplacental bleeding results in further placental detachment which may lead to fetal and maternal compromise. Haemorrhage may be concealed (20%) or revealed (80%).

INVESTIGATIONS
Bloods: FBC, clotting, U&E, X-match.
USS: Exclude placenta praevia (*note:* abruption unlikely to be evident on USS unless very large).

MANAGEMENT Depends on gestation and severity of abruption.
Mild abruption
If preterm and stable, may be managed conservatively with close monitoring; IOL if at term.

Severe abruption or maternal/fetal compromise
Requires immediate delivery by Caesarean section, airway, breathing, circulation (two large-bore IV cannulae), fluid resuscitation, correction of coagulopathy with FFP/cryoprecipitate/platelets, blood transfusion if necessary.

COMPLICATIONS
Maternal: Haemorrhage (APH + ↑ risk PPH), DIC, renal failure, 'Couvelaire' uterus (extravasation of blood into the myometrium and beneath the peritoneum).
Fetal: Birth asphyxia, death.

PROGNOSIS
Maternal: Mortality 0.5% in severe abruption.
Fetal: Mortality 3.3% in severe abruption.

Placenta praevia

DEFINITION A placenta wholly or partly inserting into the lower segment.

AETIOLOGY Unknown.

ASSOCIATIONS/RISK FACTORS Multiple pregnancy, ↑maternal age, previous uterine surgery, previous placenta praevia, smoking.

EPIDEMIOLOGY Affects 0.5% of pregnancies.

HISTORY Usually detected on routine ultrasound. Acutely, presents with painless PV bleeding in the second/third trimester.

EXAMINATION
General: May be shocked (tachycardia, hypotension)
Abdomen: Usually soft, non-tender, ?malpresentation.
Vaginal: Contraindicated.
Speculum: Gentle speculum examination permitted (assess bleeding).

PATHOLOGY/PATHOGENESIS Unknown. Abnormal implantation thought to occur where blood supply disrupted (e.g. uterine scar). Bleeding occurs secondary to shearing forces.
Minor placenta praevia: Placenta close to, but not covering, internal cervical os.
Major placenta praevia: Placenta overlying internal cervical os.

INVESTIGATIONS
Bloods: FBC, U&E, clotting, X-match.
CTG: Fetal wellbeing.
USS: Confirm placental site.
MRI: May be used to determine placenta accreta (placenta adherent to uterine wall) or placenta increta/percreta (placenta invades into or through the uterine wall).

MANAGEMENT
Vaginal delivery: Only possible if lower placental edge >2 cm from internal os and fetal head below placenta.
Caesarean section: If no bleeding, aim for 38/40.
Mild self-limiting bleed, no fetal/maternal compromise: Admit for monitoring, steroids if preterm, anti-D if Rhesus negative.
Severe bleed or fetal/maternal compromise: Manage as for severe placental abruption or maternal/fetal compromise (see above).

COMPLICATIONS
Maternal: Haemorrhage (APH + ↑ risk PPH), DIC, hysterectomy.
Fetal: IUGR, death.

PROGNOSIS Maternal mortality is 1 per 300.

Polyhydramnios

DEFINITION Increased volume of amniotic fluid, above 95th centile, or deepest pool greater than 8 cm.

AETIOLOGY Idiopathic, failure of fetal swallowing (neurological, chromosomal anomalies), fetal GI tract abnormality (duodenal/oesophageal atresia), congenital infections, fetal polyuria (diabetes, TTTS).

ASSOCIATIONS/RISK FACTORS As above.

EPIDEMIOLOGY Affects 1–4% of pregnancies.

HISTORY Symptoms of underlying aetiology, maternal discomfort.

EXAMINATION
Abdomen: ↑ fundal height, impalpable fetal parts, tense abdomen.

PATHOLOGY/PATHOGENESIS Raised amniotic fluid volume caused by increased fetal urine production or failure of fetal swallowing/intestinal absorption.

INVESTIGATIONS
USS: Diagnosis + assessment of liquor volume, fetal growth, umbilical artery Dopplers, exclude fetal anomalies.
Other: Exclude maternal diabetes.

MANAGEMENT
Amnioreduction: Only if gross polyhydramnios is causing significant discomfort.
Cyclo-oxygenase inhibitors: Occasionally used to decrease fetal urine output.
Diabetes: Optimise diabetic control.
Other: Paediatrician present at delivery.

COMPLICATIONS PTL, malpresentation, placental abruption, cord prolapse, complications of underlying pathology, PPH, ↑ risk Caesarean section.

PROGNOSIS Increased perinatal morbidity and mortality, related to PTL/congenital anomalies.

Postnatal depression

DEFINITION
Postpartum blues: Mild, self-limiting low mood in the postnatal period.
Postnatal depression: Pervasive low mood in the postnatal period.
Puerperal psychosis: Acute onset of psychotic illness in the postnatal period.

AETIOLOGY Poorly understood.

ASSOCIATIONS/RISK FACTORS Past psychiatric history, previous postnatal depression, antenatal or delivery complications, primigravidity (postnatal blues), social isolation.

EPIDEMIOLOGY
Postpartum blues: >80% of new mothers.
Postnatal depression: 10% of new mothers.
Puerperal psychosis: 1 per 1000 new mothers.

HISTORY
Postpartum blues: Emotional lability, irritability, poor sleep and concentration (often day 3–5 postnatally).
Postnatal depression: Low mood, decreased appetite, early-morning waking, anhedonia, anxiety (often occurs up to 6 weeks postnatally).
Puerperal psychosis: Mania, delusions, hallucinations, thoughts of self-harm (often presents day 3–7 postnatally).

EXAMINATION Mental state examination, depression scales may be used.

PATHOLOGY/PATHOGENESIS Poorly understood, thought to be related to falling levels of oestrogens, progesterone and cortisol postnatally.

INVESTIGATIONS NA.

MANAGEMENT
Postpartum blues: Reassurance, support (self-limiting).
Postnatal depression: Depends on severity – counselling, CBT, antidepressants.
Puerperal psychosis: Psychiatric emergency requiring inpatient admission – antidepressants, antipsychotics, ?ECT.

COMPLICATIONS Poor emotional attachment to child, long-term psychiatric morbidity, suicide (up to 5% with puerperal psychosis), infanticide (up to 4% with puerperal psychosis).

PROGNOSIS Recurrence in subsequent pregnancies: postnatal depression 30%, puerperal psychosis 20%.

Postpartum haemorrhage

DEFINITION Blood loss of >500 mL at vaginal delivery or >1000 mL at Caesarean section.

Primary PPH: Within 24 hours.
Secondary PPH: 24 hours to 6 weeks.

AETIOLOGY
Primary PPH: Uterine atony (80%), trauma to perineum/vagina/cervix, retained placenta/membranes, coagulopathy.
Secondary PPH: Endometritis, retained placenta/membranes.

ASSOCIATIONS/RISK FACTORS Multiple pregnancy, polyhydramnios, APH, grand multiparity, fibroid uterus, previous PPH, prolonged labour, augmented labour, instrumental delivery, high birthweight infant, personal or family history of bleeding disorder, anticoagulant use, Caesarean section, pyrexia in labour, episiotomy, placental site abnormalities.

EPIDEMIOLOGY Affects 5% of deliveries.

HISTORY
Primary: Excessive PV bleed after delivery (*note:* verify whether placenta is complete).
Secondary: PV bleed, abdominal pain, PV discharge, fever.

EXAMINATION
Primary
General: Shock (tachycardia, hypotension), signs of anaemia.
Abdomen: ?atonic uterus (above umbilicus)
Speculum: Exclude trauma (perineal/vaginal/cervical).
Vaginal: Evacuate clots from cervix (inhibits contraction).

Secondary
Abdomen: Tender uterus.
Speculum: Assess bleeding, ?cervical os open.
Vaginal: ?uterine tenderness.

PATHOLOGY/PATHOGENESIS See the aetiologies noted above. Placental blood flow >500 mL/min at term. With atony, poor uterine contraction (compresses spiral arteries) leads to heavy blood loss.

INVESTIGATIONS
Primary
Bloods: FBC, U&E, clotting, X-match.

Secondary
Bloods: FBC, U&E, clotting, X-match, CRP.
Microbiology: HVS.
USS: ?retained products.

MANAGEMENT
Primary
Airway, breathing, circulation (two large-bore IV cannulae), fluid resuscitation, blood transfusion if necessary.

Atony: Bimanual compression, uterotonics (oxytocin bolus + infusion, IM ergometrine, IM carboprost, PR misoprosol), transfer to theatre.
Consider: Intra-uterine balloon insertion, uterine artery embolisation, laparotomy and insertion of brace suture, hysterectomy.
Trauma: Requires suturing (consider transferring to theatre).

Postpartum haemorrhage (continued)

Retained products: Manual evacuation in theatre.
Coagulopathy: Correct with FFP/cryoprecipitate/platelets.

Secondary

Resuscitate as appropriate, IV antibiotics, ERPC only if unavoidable (increased risk of uterine perforation).

COMPLICATIONS Death, hysterectomy, ↑VTE, renal failure, DIC, Sheehan's syndrome (pituitary hypoperfusion following massive PPH causes pituitary necrosis and hypopituitarism).

PROGNOSIS Fourth most common cause of maternal death in the UK. Leading cause of maternal mortality worldwide.

Pre-eclampsia

DEFINITION Proteinuric hypertension in pregnancy, developing after 20/40.

AETIOLOGY See pathology/pathogenesis below.

ASSOCIATIONS/RISK FACTORS Nulliparity, ↑maternal age, family history, previous history of pre-eclampsia, pre-existing hypertension, new partner, pre-existing renal disease, diabetes, PCOS, multiple pregnancy, obesity.

EPIDEMIOLOGY Affects 2–5% of pregnancies.

HISTORY Headache, oedema, visual disturbance, right upper quadrant pain due to liver capsule swelling (*note:* often asymptomatic).

EXAMINATION
General: ↑BP, oedema (especially facial), hyperreflexia, clonus, ?papilloedema
Abdomen: ?RUQ tenderness, ?reduced fundal height.

PATHOLOGY/PATHOGENESIS Impaired trophoblastic invasion into the spiral arteries during placentation. Increased resistance in the uteroplacental circulation leads to hypoperfusion/ischaemia releasing inflammatory mediators which cause widespread endothelial damage, end-organ dysfunction and oedema.

INVESTIGATIONS
Bloods: FBC (↓platelets, haemoconcentration), U&E and urate (renal impairment), LFT (↑ transaminases), clotting.
Urine: Urinalysis (proteinuria), MSU (exclude UTI), 24 h urine collection (significant proteinuria >0.3 g protein per 24 hours).
USS: Fetal growth, liquor volume and umbilical artery Dopplers.
CTG: Fetal wellbeing.

MANAGEMENT Depends on gestational age and severity of condition. The condition will not resolve until after delivery.

Mild/moderate pre-eclampsia: Regular monitoring of BP with urinalysis, regular blood testing, serial USS for fetal growth, regular CTGs, antihypertensives (e.g. methyldopa, labetalol, nifedipine), aim for delivery after 37 weeks.
Severe pre-eclampsia/evidence of fetal compromise: (*Note:* requires delivery) antihypertensives (labetalol, nifedipine, hydralazine), seizure prophylaxis (IV magnesium sulphate), fluid restriction and strict fluid balance (catheterise, consider CVP monitoring), steroids for lung maturity if preterm.

COMPLICATIONS
Maternal: Eclampsia, abruption, CVA, pulmonary oedema, cerebral oedema, renal failure, liver failure, DIC, HELLP syndrome (haemolysis, elevated liver enzymes, low platelets)
Fetal: IUGR, death.

PROGNOSIS Severe pre-eclampsia has 10% recurrence in subsequent pregnancies.

Prelabour rupture of membranes (PROM) at term

DEFINITION Spontaneous rupture of membranes prior to onset of labour at term.

AETIOLOGY Natural physiological mechanisms including Braxton Hicks contractions and cervical ripening lead to weakening of the membranes.

ASSOCIATIONS/RISK FACTORS None known.

EPIDEMIOLOGY Affects 8% of pregnant women.

HISTORY Sudden gush of fluid loss PV, followed by constant trickle.

EXAMINATION
General: Assess for signs of infection (fever, tachycardia).
Vaginal: Avoid if possible (↑ risk infection).
Speculum: (If history uncertain) confirm pooling of liquor in vagina, note liquor colour.

PATHOLOGY/PATHOGENESIS NA.

INVESTIGATIONS
Microbiology: Consider HVS/LVS.

MANAGEMENT
Clear liquor and no known GBS
Expectant management for 24 hours (majority of women will labour). Offer augmentation of labour after 24 hours (may opt for expectant management for up to 72 hours with 4-hourly temperature and 24-hourly fetal monitoring). Augment labour with prostaglandin or oxytocin infusion. Antibiotic cover (benzylpenicillin or clindamycin if penicillin allergic) dependent on unit protocol.

Meconium or known GBS or pyrexia
Augment labour immediately (antibiotics if known GBS/pyrexia).

Postnatal
Neonatal observation required for at least 12 hours.

COMPLICATIONS Increased risk of ascending infection.

PROGNOSIS Sixty percent of women will labour over the next 24 hours.

Preterm prelabour rupture of membranes (PPROM)

DEFINITION Spontaneous rupture of membranes prior to onset of labour in a pregnancy <37 weeks.

AETIOLOGY Weakening of the membranes strongly linked to an infective cause (often subclinical).

ASSOCIATIONS/RISK FACTORS Also associated with APH, trauma, UTI, previous PROM/PTL, uterine abnormalities, cervical incompetence, smoking, multiple pregnancy, polyhydramnios.

EPIDEMIOLOGY Affects 2% of pregnancies.

HISTORY Sudden gush of fluid loss PV, followed by constant trickle.

EXAMINATION
General: Assess for signs of infection (fever, tachycardia).
Vaginal: Avoid (↑ risk infection)
Speculum: Confirm pooling of liquor in vagina, note liquor colour.

PATHOLOGY/PATHOGENESIS See the aetiological link noted above.

INVESTIGATIONS
Bloods: FBC, CRP (?infection)
Microbiology: MSU, HVS/LVS.
CTG: Fetal wellbeing.
USS: Confirm presentation, estimated fetal weight.

MANAGEMENT Admit for monitoring (48–72 h), steroids (fetal lung maturity), antibiotic (erythromycin 250 mg 4 × daily for 10 days), monitor temperature 4-hourly, regular CTG. Consider tocolysis in the presence of uterine activity only if intrauterine transfer required or for steroid cover. If subsequently managed as an outpatient: weekly HVS and bloods, twice daily temperature check (monitor for infection). Aim to deliver after 34/40, or earlier if evidence of infection. If <23/40, discuss TOP (extremely poor outcomes).

COMPLICATIONS
Maternal: Sepsis, placental abruption.
Fetal: Chorioamnionitis, cord prolapse, PTL, pulmonary hypoplasia, limb contractures, death.

PROGNOSIS Increased perinatal mortality predominantly due to sepsis, prematurity and pulmonary hypoplasia.

Preterm labour (PTL)

DEFINITION Onset of labour prior to 37 weeks' gestation.

AETIOLOGY May be idiopathic. Infection (often subclinical) contributes increasingly to aetiology with decreasing gestation. See pathology/pathogenesis below.

ASSOCIATIONS/RISK FACTORS Infection of genital tract, UTI, multiple pregnancy, polyhydramnios, cervical incompetence/previous cervical surgery, systemic infective illness, previous PTL, uterine abnormalities, APH.

EPIDEMIOLOGY Affects 6% of deliveries in the UK.

HISTORY Regular painful contractions, although may present as diffuse pains or cramping. ? PV bleed, ?SROM.

EXAMINATION
General: Signs of infection (tachycardia, fever).
Abdomen: Contractions, abdominal tenderness (may indicate abruption, chorioamnionitis).
Speculum: ?liquor pooling.
Vaginal: Assess cervical dilatation.

PATHOLOGY/PATHOGENESIS Relationship with systemic infective illness may be due to direct spread of infection or release of inflammatory mediators. Decidual haemorrhage is also associated with release of inflammatory mediators. PTL in polyhydramnios/multiple pregnancy is related to uterine over-distension.

INVESTIGATIONS
Bloods: FBC, CRP (evidence of infection).
Microbiology: MSU, LVS/HVS.
CTG: Fetal wellbeing.
USS: Confirm presentation, estimated fetal weight, cervical length.
Fetal fibronectin: (Sample taken at speculum examination) predictive of likelihood to labour (used for high negative predictive value).

MANAGEMENT Administer steroids (fetal lung maturation), tocolysis used to allow steroid cover e.g. oxytocin antagonists (atosiban), nifedipine or GTN (contraindicated if APH or evidence of infection), antibiotics if SROM, fetal monitoring.

COMPLICATIONS Respiratory distress syndrome, intracranial haemorrhage, sepsis, necrotising enterocolitis, neurodevelopmental delay, cerebral palsy, neonatal death.

PROGNOSIS Dependent on gestation at delivery, accounts for over 20% of perinatal mortality. There is 20% risk of PTL in subsequent pregnancies.

Prolonged labour

DEFINITION Poor progress in labour.

First stage
Primip: Cervical dilatation of less than 2 cm in 4 hours.
Multip: Cervical dilatation of less than 2 cm in 4 hours or a slowing in progress.

Second stage
A delay in delivery of >2 h (primp) or >1 h (multip) from active pushing.

Third stage
Failure to deliver the placenta after >30 min (active management), >1 h (physiological). *See* National Institute for Health and Clinical Excellence clinical guideline, *Intrapartum Care: Management and Delivery of Care to Women in Labour*, 2007.

AETIOLOGY
First/second stage
'Powers': Frequency and duration of contractions.
'Passenger': Fetal size, malpresentation, malpositioning.
'Passages': CPD.

Third stage
Failure of the placenta to detach from the placental bed.

ASSOCIATIONS/RISK FACTORS
First/second stage
See the aetiologies noted above. *Also:* primigravidity, ↑maternal age, big baby, short stature, obesity, induction of labour, epidural (delay in second stage), cervical surgery, pelvic trauma, fetal malformations.

Third stage
Previous retained placenta, previous injury to uterus, pre-term delivery, induction of labour, multiparity.

EPIDEMIOLOGY
First/second stage
Contributes to 30–50% of overall Caesarean section rates.

Third stage
Affects 0.8–1.2% of births.

HISTORY Assess risk factors as above, review partogram.

EXAMINATION
First/second stage
General: Maternal exhaustion, dehydration, blood-stained urine (sign of obstructed labour).
Abdomen: Fetal size, lie, presentation, engagement.
Vaginal: Cervical dilatation, station, presentation, position, presence of membranes, signs of obstruction (caput/moulding), assess pelvic capacity.

Third stage
Failure of placental delivery with controlled cord traction.

PATHOLOGY/PATHOGENESIS See the aetiologies noted above.

INVESTIGATIONS
Bloods: FBC, G&S (preparation for delivery/theatre).
CTG: Fetal wellbeing (first/second stage).

Prolonged labour (continued)

MANAGEMENT
First stage
Fluid rehydration, adequate pain relief, ARM if appropriate, augmentation of labour with oxytocin infusion (caution in multips). Caesarean section for malpresentation. Consider FBS/delivery if signs of fetal distress.

Second stage
Consider oxytocin. If fully dilated, <1/5 palpable abdominally and vertex at/below spines: instrumental delivery. Otherwise Caesarean section.

Third stage
Administer oxytocin, if still retained after 30 minutes needs manual removal of placenta (often in theatre).

COMPLICATIONS
First/second stage
Maternal: Risks of instrumental delivery or Caesarean section, PPH, uterine rupture, fistula formation (rare in UK).
Fetal: Fetal distress, complications of instrumental delivery, ↑ risk shoulder dystocia.

Third stage
PPH, infection.

PROGNOSIS
First/second stage
While many cases respond to intervention, prolonged labour still accounts for a high proportion of Caesareans.

Third stage
Good prognosis.

Prolonged pregnancy

DEFINITION Pregnancy that proceeds beyond 42 weeks.

AETIOLOGY Unknown.

ASSOCIATIONS/RISK FACTORS Previous post-term pregnancy, primiparity, obesity.

EPIDEMIOLOGY Affects 5–15% of pregnancies.

HISTORY Failure to enter spontaneous labour by 42 weeks. Ensure adequate fetal movements and accurate dating from early USS.

EXAMINATION
Abdomen: Fundal height, auscultate FH.
Vaginal: Assess cervix for induction of labour.

PATHOLOGY/PATHOGENESIS Placental function decreases post-term (histology shows calcification, syncytial knotting), associated with increased rates of perinatal morbidity and mortality.

INVESTIGATIONS
USS: Liquor volume, growth.
CTG: At least twice-weekly for fetal wellbeing.

MANAGEMENT All women should be offered membrane sweeping from 40–41/40 (↑ likelihood spontaneous labour). Induction of labour should be offered at between 41 and 42 weeks. Women's decisions to decline induction should be respected, but they should be advised that no monitoring techniques are predictive of fetal death.

COMPLICATIONS Increased risk of stillbirth (from 1 per 1000 at 37/40 to 3 per 1000 at 42/40), ↑ risk perinatal morbidity/mortality, ↑ risk Caesarean section, ↑ meconium staining of liquor.

PROGNOSIS Recurrence of 30% in subsequent pregnancies.

Rhesus isoimmunisation

DEFINITION Development of Rhesus antibodies in a Rhesus-negative mother after exposure to Rhesus-positive blood cells (most commonly RhD antigen).

AETIOLOGY A sensitising event exposes a RhD-negative mother to a RhD-positive fetus' red blood cells (can occur through RhD-positive blood transfusion but rare in the UK). Maternal antibodies develop to RhD. In subsequent pregnancies involving a RhD-positive fetus, maternal IgG antibodies will cross the placenta, forming complexes with RhD on fetal erythrocytes and destroying them. Sensitising events include delivery, APH, miscarriage, ectopic pregnancy, TOP and invasive prenatal testing.

ASSOCIATIONS/RISK FACTORS Previous pregnancy with insufficient/without anti-D prophylaxis, previous blood transfusion (rare if occurred in the UK).

EPIDEMIOLOGY Fifteen percent of Caucasian populations are RhD-negative. Without prophylaxis, isoimmunisation occurs in 1%.

HISTORY Often picked up on routine antenatal screening, patient may be aware of diagnosis from previous pregnancies. May have poor obstetric history.

EXAMINATION NA.

PATHOLOGY/PATHOGENESIS IgG antibodies against RhD-positive fetal red cells cause haemolysis leading to anaemia, hyperbilirubinaemia and subsequent hydrops fetalis (fetal heart failure associated with accumulation of fluid subcutaneously and in body compartments – e.g. ascites, pericardial effusion).

INVESTIGATIONS Regular monitoring of maternal antibody levels. Once threshold level for prediction of anaemia is reached, needs monitoring in a fetal medicine centre with USS markers of anaemia (e.g. MCA Doppler). Monitoring may also include: measurement of amniotic fluid bilirubin concentration, or cordocentesis.

MANAGEMENT

Prevention: Anti-D immunoglobulin prophylaxis is recommended for all RhD-negative mothers at 28/40 and 34/40, following any sensitising event, and after delivery (if baby is RhD-positive).

Rhesus isoimmunisation in current pregnancy: May necessitate fetal blood transfusions during pregnancy, and exchange transfusion in the neonate following delivery.

COMPLICATIONS Hydrops fetalis, intrauterine death, neonatal death, neonatal kernicterus.

PROGNOSIS Dependent on the severity of disease.

Shoulder dystocia

DEFINITION Difficulty with delivering the fetal shoulders following delivery of the head.

AETIOLOGY Bony impaction of the anterior fetal shoulder behind the maternal symphysis pubis.

ASSOCIATIONS/RISK FACTORS High birthweight baby (although 50% occur with normal birthweight babies), post-dates, previous shoulder dystocia, diabetes, obesity, instrumental delivery, prolonged labour.

EPIDEMIOLOGY Affects 1% of deliveries.

HISTORY Delay in delivery of fetal shoulders, 'turtle-necking' of fetal head.

EXAMINATION Evidence of shoulder dystocia as above.

PATHOLOGY/PATHOGENESIS NA.

INVESTIGATIONS NA.

MANAGEMENT The mnemonic HELPERR below is often used. Each manoeuvre should be attempted for up to 30 seconds. Meticulous documentation is mandatory.
H: Call for help.
E: Evaluate for episiotomy.
L: Legs – the McRoberts manoeuvre, hyperflexing the maternal thighs on to the abdomen.
P: Pressure suprapubically on to the posterior aspect of the fetal shoulder.
E: Enter manoeuvres – for internal rotation of the fetal shoulders into the oblique plane.
R: Remove the posterior arm.
R: Roll the patient on to all-fours.

Manoeuvres of last resort include deliberate clavicular fracture, symphysiotomy, general anaesthesia and the Zavanelli manoeuvre (replacement of the fetal head followed by Caesarean section).

COMPLICATIONS
Maternal: PPH, uterine rupture, extensive perineal tears (↑ third/fourth degree tears), symphyseal separation.
Fetal: Death, hypoxic–ischaemic encephalopathy, fractured humerus/clavicle, brachial plexus injury.

PROGNOSIS Perinatal mortality is 1–2%. A quarter of infants suffer brachial plexus injury (1–2% long-term dysfunction). 10–15% recurrence in future pregnancies.

Venous thromboembolism (VTE) in pregnancy

DEFINITION
Deep vein thrombosis (DVT): Formation of blood clot in deep veins (usually of the leg).
Pulmonary embolism (PE): Distal spread of a thrombus to the pulmonary vasculature.

AETIOLOGY Thrombus formation initiated by endothelial injury/stasis/hypercoagulability
(Virchow's triad). Commonly occurs in deep veins of leg/pelvis and embolises to pulmonary
vasculature. Pregnancy is a pro-coagulant state.

ASSOCIATIONS/RISK FACTORS
General: ↑maternal age, thrombophilia, obesity, personal or family history of PE, smoking,
   immobility, post-surgery.
Pregnancy: Caesarean section (especially emergency), instrumental delivery, infection,
   pre-eclampsia, multiple pregnancy, hyperemesis/dehydration.

EPIDEMIOLOGY Affects 1 per 6000 pregnancies.

HISTORY
DVT: Classically red, hot, swollen tender calf.
PE: Pleuritic chest pain, dyspnoea, cough, haemoptysis.

EXAMINATION
Deep vein thrombosis
Unilateral lower limb oedema, erythema, tenderness, may have low-grade pyrexia.

Pulmonary embolism
General: Tachycardia, tachypnoea, low-grade pyrexia, reduced O_2 saturation on pulse
   oximetry, cardiorespiratory collapse (rare).
Chest auscultation: May be normal or reveal reduced air entry, crepitations.
Cardiovascular: ?loud P2.

PATHOLOGY/PATHOGENESIS See the aetiologies noted above.

INVESTIGATIONS
Deep vein thrombosis
Duplex USS.

Pulmonary embolism
General: ABG (hypoxia/hypocapnia), ECG (sinus tachycardia/S1Q3T3).
Imaging: CXR, duplex USS (if both negative, then V/Q or CTPA).
Bloods: (Prior to anticoagulation) FBC, U&E, LFT, clotting.

MANAGEMENT
Prevention: All obstetric patients should be evaluated for thromboprophylaxis (e.g.
   compression stockings, LMWH).
Treatment: LMWH, initiated on clinical suspicion and discontinued if diagnosis excluded.
   Continue for remainder of pregnancy. Discontinue at start of labour or 24 hours prior to
   planned delivery. Continue treatment 6/52 postnatally (can convert to PO anticoagulation
   3/7 after delivery).
Massive PE: ABC, multidisciplinary management, IV unfractionated heparin preferred. May
   rarely require thrombolysis, thoracotomy or surgical embolectomy.

COMPLICATIONS Death, effects of long-term anticoagulation, post-thrombotic leg
syndrome.

PROGNOSIS Pulmonary embolism is the largest single cause of maternal death in the UK,
resulting in 15 maternal deaths/year.

Gynaecology

Amenorrhoea

DEFINITION

Primary amenorrhoea: Failure to establish menstruation by the age of 16 years or by 14 years of age if no secondary sexual characteristics.

Secondary amenorrhoea: Absence of menstruation for $\geq$6 consecutive months in a woman who has previously established regular menses.

AETIOLOGY

Primary amenorrhoea (5%)

Normal secondary sexual characteristics: Constitutional delay (most common), androgen insensitivity syndrome, anatomical defects (imperforate hymen, transverse vaginal septum, absent vagina ± non-functioning uterus).

Absent secondary sexual characteristics: Kallman's syndrome, anorexia nervosa, excessive exercise, gonadal agenesis (46XX/46XY), gonadal dysgenesis (e.g. Turner syndrome – 45X), congenital infections, pituitary tumours, head injury, cranial irradiation.

Intersex conditions: CAH, 5α reductase deficiency, true hermaphrodites.

Secondary amenorrhoea (95%)

Pregnancy: Most common cause (always consider).

Ovary (60% of pathological causes): PCOS (35%), premature ovarian failure (25%).

Pituitary: Hypopituitarism, Sheehan's syndrome, trauma, tumour (e.g. prolactinoma), cranial irradiation.

Hypothalamus: Hypogonadotrophic hypogonadism (extreme exercise, ↓ weight, idiopathic or chronic illness may result in thalamic suppression).

Uterine (rare): Asherman's syndrome, cervical stenosis

Others: Endocrine (thyroid disease, Cushing's).

ASSOCIATIONS/RISK FACTORS See the aetiologies noted above.

EPIDEMIOLOGY Prevalence: primary 0.5%, secondary 3–5%.

HISTORY LMP, menarche, previous menstrual history, medications (incl. contraceptive use), development history/height (primary), weight change, exercise, recent/chronic illness, symptoms of climacteric, hirsutism, acne, symptoms of other endocrine disorder, galactorrhoea, visual change.

EXAMINATION

Primary: Assess stature, secondary sexual characteristics, assess anatomical abnormalities (e.g. imperforate hymen).

Secondary: Weight (↑ or ↓), ?hirsutism, alopecia, acne, visual fields (pituitary tumour), signs of other endocrine dysfunction, ?vaginal atrophy.

PATHOLOGY/PATHOGENESIS Dependent on the aetiology.

INVESTIGATIONS

Primary amenorrhoea

Bloods: LH, FSH, oestradiol, prolactin, ?karyotype.

Imaging: Pelvic ultrasound.

Secondary amenorrhoea

Bloods: LH, FSH, oestradiol, prolactin, testosterone, androstenedione, SHBG, TFT, ?ACTH stimulation test/dexamethasone suppression test (if other endocrine pathology suspected).

Imaging: USS pelvis, HSG (if ?Asherman's), MRI pituitary fossa (if ↑ prolactin).

Other: Bone mineral density scan (if oestrogen deficiency), urinary β-HCG (exclude pregnancy), hysteroscopy (if ?Asherman's).

Amenorrhoea (continued)

MANAGEMENT

Primary amenorrhoea

Constitutional delay: Conservative.

Other (dependent on aetiology): May require surgical correction of anatomical abnormality, surgical reconstruction, psychological counselling, gender assignment, gonadectomy (↑ malignancy 46XY), bromocriptine (prolactinoma), treatment for eating disorder, hormone replacement.

Secondary amenorrhoea

Dependent on cause. May require HRT (premature ovarian failure), management of PCOS (see Polycystic ovarian syndrome), surgical treatment of Asherman's, bromocriptine (prolactinoma), weight management, treatment of other endocrine cause (e.g. thyroxine replacement).

COMPLICATIONS Osteoporosis if oestrogen deficiency, endometrial hyperplasia/malignancy (PCOS), infertility. Karyotypic abnormalities and disorders of intersex may have profound psychological implications.

PROGNOSIS Dependent on the aetiology.

Asherman's syndrome

DEFINITION Presence of intrauterine adhesions that may partially or completely occlude the uterine cavity.

AETIOLOGY Damage to the endometrium involving the basal layer, owing to factors such as trauma (from instrumentation) or infection. Leads to fibrosis and adhesion formation.

ASSOCIATIONS/RISK FACTORS Endometrial resection, excessive curettage (e.g. following miscarriage, TOP), surgery (myomectomy, Caesarean section), endometritis.

EPIDEMIOLOGY Uncommon although incidence and prevalence vary widely.

HISTORY Menstrual disturbance (often amenorrhoea), cyclical abdominal pain, subfertility.

EXAMINATION No external physical signs.

PATHOLOGY/PATHOGENESIS Adhesions may be filmy consisting of basal endometrium, *or* fibromuscular covered by endometrium, *or* entirely composed of connective tissue.

INVESTIGATIONS
Imaging: HSG (radiological filling defects), saline hysterosonography.
Other: Hysteroscopy.

MANAGEMENT
Surgical: Hysteroscopic adhesiolysis (myometrial scoring may increase cavity dimensions in severely narrowed cavities).
Post-procedure: Copper IUCD placed in cavity to prevent adhesion formation, PO oestrogens (induce endometrial proliferation), reassess cavity 2–3 months after treatment.

COMPLICATIONS Infertility, miscarriage, menstrual disturbance, abnormal placentation in future pregnancies, complications of operative treatment.

PROGNOSIS Menstrual disturbance often improves after treatment. Post-treatment pregnancy rates of 50% are reported (although increased complication rates).

Atrophic vaginitis

DEFINITION Vaginal irritation caused by thinning of the vaginal epithelium.

AETIOLOGY Caused by a reduction in circulating oestrogen levels.

ASSOCIATIONS/RISK FACTORS Menopause, prolonged lactation.

EPIDEMIOLOGY True prevalence unknown, ? 10–40% of postmenopausal women.

HISTORY Vaginal irritation, dyspareunia, superficial dysuria, discharge (may be bloodstained).

EXAMINATION Pale, thin vaginal walls with loss of rugal folds, ?cracks/fissures.

PATHOLOGY/PATHOGENESIS Reduced circulating oestrogens leads to loss of glycogen in epithelial cells and ↑ vaginal pH.

INVESTIGATIONS Swabs may be taken for superimposed infection. Any suspicious lesions warrant exclusion of malignancy. Presentation with bleeding may necessitate investigation as per PMB.

MANAGEMENT Systemic HRT or topical oestrogens.

COMPLICATIONS Increased incidence of superinfection due to ↑ vaginal pH.

PROGNOSIS Substantial relief can be achieved with treatment.

Bartholin's cyst/abscess

DEFINITION Cyst or abscess of the Bartholin's gland.

AETIOLOGY Obstruction of the Bartholin's duct leads to accumulation of fluid and distension of the gland.

ASSOCIATIONS/RISK FACTORS Generally occur in women aged 20–30 years.

EPIDEMIOLOGY Affects 2% of women of reproductive age.

HISTORY Unilateral vulval swelling. *Cyst*: often painless. *Abscess*: pain, difficulty walking/ sitting, dyspareunia.

EXAMINATION Unilateral swelling in region of Bartholin's gland. Abscess will be tender, fluctuant, warm, erythematous, surrounding cellulitis.

PATHOLOGY/PATHOGENESIS Superinfection now predominantly caused by *Streptococcus*, *Staphylococcus* and *E. coli* (previously *C. trachomatis* and *N. gonorrhoeae*).

INVESTIGATIONS
Microbiology: Cyst fluid/cavity swab for MC&S.

MANAGEMENT
Small painless cysts: Conservative treatment.
Small abscesses: May respond to antibiotics.
Large abscesses: Require marsupialisation (incision of the gland and formation of a tract from the interior wall of the cyst to the exterior).

COMPLICATIONS Recurrence.

PROGNOSIS Recurrence rate of 20%.

Benign ovarian mass

DEFINITION Non-malignant tumour of the ovary: epithelial (e.g. Brenner's tumour, mucinous adenoma, serous adenoma), sex-cord stromal tumour (e.g. fibroma, thecoma), germ-cell (e.g. mature cystic teratoma), endometrioma, functional (follicular, luteal, haemorrhagic).

AETIOLOGY Largely unknown. Endometriomas result from endometriosis. Functional cysts form around ovulation. Cyst accidents are caused by cyst rupture, haemorrhage into a cyst, or torsion (rotation of the ovary on its pedicle – risk of ischaemia and necrosis).

ASSOCIATIONS/RISK FACTORS Unclear except for endometriosis (endometriomas).

EPIDEMIOLOGY Four percent of women have hospital attendances with ovarian cysts prior to age 65.

HISTORY Lower abdominal pain, deep dyspareunia, pressure symptoms, abdominal swelling (*note:* may be asymptomatic).
Acute accident: Severe right or left iliac fossa pain, accompanied by vomiting in torsion.

EXAMINATION
Abdomen: Iliac fossa tenderness, rebound/guarding with acute accident.
Vaginal: Adnexal tenderness ± palpable mass.

PATHOLOGY/PATHOGENESIS
Epithelial
Serous cystadenoma: Most common epithelial tumour – thin-walled, often uniloculated, filled with watery fluid, lined by cuboidal epithelium.
Mucinous cystadenoma: Usually large, unilateral, multiloculated, filled with thick fluid, lined by mucous-secreting columnar cells.
Brenner's: Rare solid pale yellow tumour, contains nests of transitional epithelium.

Sex-cord stromal
Thecoma: Solid yellow tumour, lipid filled cells, typically oestrogen-secreting.
Fibroma: Solid white tumour (+ ascites and pleural effusion → Meig's syndrome).

Mature cystic teratoma (dermoid)
Derived from germ cells, therefore may contain ectodermal tissue (squamous epithelium, teeth, hair, sebaceous glands), endodermal tissue (thyroid, intestine) or mesodermal tissue (cartilage). 10% are bilateral.

Endometrioma
Retention cysts due to endometriosis.

Functional cysts
Follicular: Unruptured Graafian follicle (failed rupture of dominant follicle/failure of non-dominant to degenerate), lined by granulosa cells.
Luteal: Following rupture, follicle reseals and distends with fluid – lined by luteal cells.
Haemorrhagic: Bleeding into a functional cyst.

INVESTIGATIONS
Acute presentation: Investigation should proceed as per any acute abdominal pain including exclusion of pregnancy.
USS: Diagnostic (TVS preferable).
Bloods: FBC, G&S (preparation for theatre), tumour markers (Ca 125, HCG, AFP).

MANAGEMENT
Small simple cysts
Conservative, repeat scan at 3–6 months.

Benign ovarian mass (continued)

Suspicion of torsion, or cysts >5 cm

Ovarian cystectomy (laparoscopic/open), oophorectomy if surgical difficulty/necrosis/ suspicious appearance – oophorectomy recommended if postmenopausal.

COMPLICATIONS Cyst accident, subfertility, malignant change, oophorectomy.

PROGNOSIS Surgery usually curative.

Carcinoma of the cervix

DEFINITION Malignancy of the uterine cervix.

AETIOLOGY HPV implicated in over 95% of cases, HPV 16 and 18 predominate.

ASSOCIATIONS/RISK FACTORS Smoking, multiple sexual partners, ↓ age at first intercourse, ↓ socioeconomic status, HIV.

EPIDEMIOLOGY Accounts for 6% of female malignancies, global incidence 500 000 new cases/year (UK: 2221 new cases in 2004).

HISTORY PV discharge (?offensive/bloodstained), PCB/IMB/PMB (*note:* may be asymptomatic, detected on screening. Late symptoms (from metastasis): lower limb oedema, haematuria, rectal bleeding, signs of fistulae, pressure symptoms.

EXAMINATION May be unremarkable if early stage/within endocervical canal.
Chest: ?signs of pulmonary metastases.
Abdomen: Masses (if pelvic spread), ?hepatomegaly.
Speculum: Discolouration, ulceration, erosion or macroscopic tumour on cervix.
Vaginal: masses (if pelvic spread).

PATHOLOGY/PATHOGENESIS
Histology: 85% squamous and adenosquamous carcinomas, 15% adenocarcinoma.
Spread: Direct or lymphatic.
Staging: (FIGO 2009) **stage Ia** – invasive carcinoma diagnosed only by microscopy (**Ia1** – stromal invasion ≤3.0 mm, extension ≤7.0 mm; **Ia2** – stromal invasion >3 mm and <5 mm, extension ≤7.0 mm); **stage Ib** – clinically visible lesions limited to the cervix, or preclinical cancers greater than stage Ia (**Ib1** – ≤4 cm; **Ib2** – >4 cm); **stage II** – invades beyond the uterus, but not to the pelvic wall or lower 1/3 of the vagina; **IIa** – without parametrial invasion (**IIa1** ≤4.0 cm; **IIa2** >4 cm); **IIb** – obvious parametrial invasion; **stage III** – extends to lower 1/3 of the vagina (**IIIa**), or extends to pelvic side wall and/or causes hydronephrosis/non-functioning kidney (**IIIb**); **stage IV** – spread beyond the true pelvis or to bladder/rectal mucosa (**IVa** adjuvent organs; **IVb** distant organs).

INVESTIGATIONS
Tissue diagnosis: Colposcopy and biopsy.
Bloods: FBC (?anaemia), U&E (?obstruction), LFT (?metastases), clotting (if LFT abnormal), G&S (surgical preparation).
Imaging: CXR, CT (radiological staging), MRI (↑accuracy, allows assessment of lymph nodes).
Other: Cystoscopy.

MANAGEMENT
Surgical
Stage I: Ia1 – cone biopsy or simple abdominal hysterectomy; Ia2 – simple hysterectomy with pelvic lymphadenectomy.
Stage Ib–IIa: Radical hysterectomy and pelvic lymphadenectomy.
Selected Ib: May be suitable for trachelectomy (radical excision of the cervix) to conserve fertility.

Chemoradiation
Stage IIb and above. External-beam radiation/brachytherapy combined with cisplatin-based therapy.

Recurrence
Consider radiation if not already given or pelvic exenteration.

Carcinoma of the cervix (continued)

COMPLICATIONS

From metastasis: Lower limb oedema, genitourinary obstruction, fistula formation.

From surgery: Bleeding, infection, urinary dysfunction (detrusor denervation), fistulae, lymphoedema.

From radiotherapy: Cystitis, rectal/vaginal stenosis, fistulae, bowel obstruction.

PROGNOSIS Five-year survival: stage I, 90–95%; stage II, 65%; stage III, 35%.

Carcinoma of the endometrium

DEFINITION Malignancy arising from the endometrial tissue.

AETIOLOGY Exact aetiology unclear, but it involves unopposed oestrogen stimulation of the endometrium.

ASSOCIATIONS/RISK FACTORS Unopposed oestrogen stimulation of endometrium.
Exogenous: Oestrogen-only HRT, tamoxifen.
Endogenous: Nulliparity/infertility (↑ number anovulatory cycles), early menarche/late menopause (also related to anovulatory cycles), PCOS, oestrogen-producing ovarian tumours (granulosa/theca), obesity (aromatisation of fat-derived peripheral androgens).
Other: Hereditary non-polyposis colon cancer (HNPCC).

EPIDEMIOLOGY Second most common gynaecological malignancy in the UK, lifetime risk 1% (*note:* uncommon under age 40 years).

HISTORY PMB, menorrhagia/IMB (if premenopausal), PV discharge (?offensive).

EXAMINATION Likely to be normal unless advanced. May have bulky uterus on bimanual.

PATHOLOGY/PATHOGENESIS
Histology: 80% endometrioid adenocarcinoma, 20% uterine papillary serous, mucinous, clear cell, squamous cell or mixed. Endometrial hyperplasia with atypia is considered premalignant.
Spread: Direct and lymphatic (haematogenous occurs late).
Staging: (FIGO 2009) **stage I** – confined to uterus; **Ia** – no or <50% myometrial invasion; **Ib** – ≤50% myometrium; **stage II** – invades cervical stroma but does not extend beyond uterus; **stage III** – local or regional spread; **IIIa** – serosa/adnexa; **IIIb** – vagina/parametrium; **IIIc** – pelvic (**IIIc1**) or para-aortic (**IIIc2**) lymph nodes; **stage IV** – invades bladder and/or bowel mucosa (**IVa**) or distant metastases (**IVb**).

INVESTIGATIONS
Tissue diagnosis: Pipelle biopsy/hysteroscopy and biopsy.
Bloods: FBC (anaemia), U&E, LFT, G&S.
Imaging: Pelvic USS (thickened endometrium, investigate if >4 mm in postmenopausal women), TVS can assess depth myometrial invasion, MRI (stage, depth myometrial invasion, pelvic lymphadenopathy), CXR (metastasis).

MANAGEMENT
Surgery: Stage I: TAH/BSO (with peritoneal washings); stage II/III: modified radical/radical hysterectomy.
Radiotherapy: As adjuvant for stage II and above (advanced disease, in combination with surgery or alone if surgery inappropriate) – external-beam and vault brachytherapy.
Chemotherapy: Limited use for palliation not amenable to radiotherapy.

COMPLICATIONS Metastatic spread, surgical morbidity, complications from radiotherapy (especially bowel)

PROGNOSIS Five-year survival: stage I 80–90%, stage II 67–77%, stage III 32–60%.

Carcinoma of the ovary

DEFINITION Malignant neoplasm of the ovary.

AETIOLOGY Exact aetiology unknown: ?increased number ovulatory cycles (?abnormal repair of ovarian surface), BRCA1 gene associated with breast–ovarian cancer syndrome.

ASSOCIATIONS/RISK FACTORS Nulliparity, ↑ age, history of fertility treatment, family history, history of breast cancer, high-fat diet, HNPCC.
Protective factors: Parity, oral contraceptive use, breastfeeding, hysterectomy.

EPIDEMIOLOGY Most common gynaecological malignancy in the UK (5% female cancers): 12.9–15.1 cases per 100 000 people, 1 in 70 lifetime risk.

HISTORY Often late presentation. Vague early symptoms: abdominal discomfort, abdominal distension/mass, fatigue, weight loss, pressure symptoms (urinary frequency/dyspepsia).

EXAMINATION
General: Signs of malignancy (anaemia, cachexia etc.).
Chest: Signs of metastasis, pleural effusion.
Abdomen: Abdominal/pelvic mass, ascites, hepatomegaly.
Pelvis: Pelvic mass.

PATHOLOGY/PATHOGENESIS Multiple histological types including:

Epithelial tumours (>90%): Include serous cystadenocarcinoma (most common, fluid-filled cystic components), mucinous cystadenocarcinoma (mucin-filled cysts), endometrioid carcinoma (resembles endometrial adenocarcinoma), clear cell carcinoma (cells have clear cytoplasm).
Germ cell tumours (<5%): Dysgerminoma most common.
Sex-cord stromal tumours (rarely malignant): Most common granulosa cell tumour.

INVESTIGATIONS
Bloods: FBC (?anaemia), U&E (obstruction, renal failure), LFT (liver metastasis, ↓ albumin/ total protein), clotting (if LFTs abnormal), tumour markers (Ca 125, HCG, AFP, CEA, Ca 15-3, Ca 19-9).
Imaging: TVS (↑ suspicion if solid areas, septae, thickened walls), MRI (for surgical planning).

MANAGEMENT
Staging laparotomy: TAH/BSO, peritoneal washings, omentectomy, peritoneal biopsies, assessment of pelvic/para-aortic lymph nodes.
Advanced disease: Debulking procedure (TAH/BSO, omentectomy, resection of metastases).
Chemotherapy: Includes platinum compounds and taxanes.
Radiotherapy: Primarily for palliation.

COMPLICATIONS Ovarian cyst accident, metastatic spread, surgical morbidity, complications of chemotherapy (bone marrow suppression, infection, nephrotoxicity), ascites, pleural effusion.

PROGNOSIS Five-year survival: stage I 80–100%, stage III 15–20%, stage IV 5%. Overall survival low owing to late-stage at presentation.

Carcinoma of the vulva

DEFINITION Malignant neoplasm of the vulva.

AETIOLOGY Progression of certain vulval dermatoses, or progression of VIN (HPV-associated).

ASSOCIATIONS/RISK FACTORS VIN, lichen sclerosis (1–2% progression), smoking.

EPIDEMIOLOGY Rare: 800 new cases per year in the UK, primarily in the elderly but also seen in premenopausal women (often HPV-associated).

HISTORY Vulval swelling/ulcer, pruritis, pain, bleeding, discharge.

EXAMINATION Nodule or ulcer visible on vulva (most commonly labia majora), ?inguinal lymphadenopathy.

PATHOLOGY/PATHOGENESIS

Histology: Majority are squamous cell, melanoma and basal cell less frequent, adenocarcinoma rare.

Spread: Direct and lymphatic.

Staging: (FIGO 2009) **stage I** – confined to vulva/perineum, negative nodes; **Ia** – ≥ 2 cm in size, stromal invasion ≥ 1.0 mm; **Ib** – >2 cm in size or stromal invasion >1.0 cm; **stage II** – tumour of any size with extension to lower 1/3 of urethra, lower 1/3 vagina or anus, with negative nodes; **stage III** – tumour of any size $\pm$ extension to lower 1/3 urethra, lower 1/3 vagina or anus with positive inguino-femoral lymph nodes and distant spread; **stage IV** – other regional or distant spread; **IVa** – (i) invading upper urethral and/or vaginal mucosa, bladder mucosa or rectal mucosa, or fixed to pelvic bone, or (ii) fixed or ulcerated inguino-femoral lymph nodes; **IVb** – distant metastases including pelvic lymph nodes.

INVESTIGATIONS

Tissue diagnosis: Full-thickness biopsy, ?sentinel node biopsy.

Cervical smear: Exclude CIN if VIN-associated.

Bloods: FBC, U&E.

Imaging: CT/MRI (assess lymphadenopathy), CXR (metastases).

Other: Staging by cystoscopy, proctoscopy.

MANAGEMENT

Surgery for early-stage disease: Wide radical local excision to reduce surgical morbidity. Ipsilateral or bilateral inguino-femoral lymph node dissection dependent on site and size of tumour. Large/multifocal lesions: radical vulvectomy.

Large/multifocal lesions: Radical vulvectomy, ?ipsilateral or bilateral inguinofemoral lymph node dissection dependent on site and size of tumour.

Radiotherapy: External-beam radiation (advanced disease/↑ risk relapse in early disease).

COMPLICATIONS Psychosexual, surgical morbidity (especially wound infection/breakdown), lower limb lymphoedema (from lymph node dissection).

PROGNOSIS Five-year survival: stage I 85–90%, with nodal involvement 50–60%.

Cervical intraepithelial neoplasia

DEFINITION Premalignant cellular atypia within the squamous epithelium of the cervix.

AETIOLOGY HPV implicated in >95% cases, HPV 16 and 18 predominate.

ASSOCIATIONS/RISK FACTORS Smoking, multiple sexual partners, ↓ age at first intercourse, ↓ socioeconomic status, HIV.

EPIDEMIOLOGY Peak incidence at 25–29 years, difficult to assess UK prevalence (only CIN3 recorded in cancer registries).

HISTORY Asymptomatic, detected on cervical screening.

EXAMINATION
Speculum: Cervix often unremarkable.

PATHOLOGY/PATHOGENESIS
Histology: Dysplastic epithelial changes – ↑nuclear-to-cytoplasmic ratio, ↑nuclear size, abnormal nuclear shape (poikilocytosis), ↑nuclear density (koilocytosis), ↓ cytoplasm.
CIN grades: **CIN I** – mild dysplasia confined to lower third of the epithelium; **CIN II** – moderate dysplasia affecting two-thirds of the epithelial thickness; **CIN III** – severe dysplasia extending to upper third of epithelium (carcinoma-in-situ). CIN I is referred to as *low-grade*, CIN II and III as *high-grade*.

INVESTIGATIONS Colposcopy ± biopsy.

MANAGEMENT
CIN I: Conservative (may resolve), but if persistent may require excision/cryotherapy (differing opinions on timing of intervention).
CIN II or III: LLETZ, conisation, laser (if family is completed/older age, consider TAH).
Follow-up: Dependent on unit and extent of disease. If smears are negative:
  CIN I: Follow-up at 6 and 18 months, then return to screening programme.
  CIN II or III: Follow-up at 6, 12 and 18 months, then annual smears for 10 years.

COMPLICATIONS Progression to cervical carcinoma. Complications of treatment are bleeding, infection, evidence of future cervical incompetence with excision procedures.

PROGNOSIS
CIN I: 20% progression to higher stages, 50% regression.
CIN II: 33% progression, 33% regression.
CIN III: 20–30% 10-year progression to carcinoma (cervical screening prevents up to 3900 cases of cervical cancer per year).

Detrusor overactivity

DEFINITION Urodynamic observation characterised by involuntary detrusor contractions (provoked or unprovoked) during the filling phase. Indicative of overactive bladder syndrome.

AETIOLOGY Idiopathic, neuropathic (e.g. multiple sclerosis), consequence of incontinence surgery.

ASSOCIATIONS/RISK FACTORS Increasing age, previous incontinence surgery, neurological disorders (e.g. MS, spinal cord injury, bladder outlet obstruction).

EPIDEMIOLOGY Accounts for 30–50% of female urinary incontinence (up to 80% in the elderly).

HISTORY Urinary urgency, urinary frequency (>8 voids/24 h), urge incontinence, nocturia. Consider use of a frequency/volume chart (records volume of fluids consumed, urine passed and episodes of urgency or incontinence).

EXAMINATION
Abdomen: Look for other causes of urgency/frequency (e.g. mass).
Vaginal: Observe for atrophy, prolapse, evidence concomitant stress incontinence.
CNS: If suspected neurological aetiology.

PATHOLOGY/PATHOGENESIS Unclear, may be related to changes in functional innervation of the bladder wall.

INVESTIGATIONS
Micro: Urine MC&S (exclude infection).
Urodynamic studies: (Only indicated if mixed symptoms, suspected voiding disorder or previous continence surgery) involuntary detrusor contraction during filling.
Other: Occasionally pelvic imaging/cystoscopy (differentials for urgency, e.g. pelvic mass, interstitial cystitis).

MANAGEMENT
Lifestyle: ↓ caffeine/alcohol intake.
Bladder training: Set voiding intervals that are lengthened when patient remains dry.
Medication: Anticholinergics – tolterodine, solifenacin, tropsium chloride, oxybutinin, propiverine.
Surgical: (Extremely rare for intractable cases) urinary diversion techniques (e.g. ileocystoplasy).

COMPLICATIONS Severe social and psychological difficulties, ↓ skin integrity (persistent contact with urine).

PROGNOSIS No cure, but significant alleviation of symptoms can be achieved with treatment. May still impact heavily on activities of daily living.

Dysfunctional uterine bleeding

DEFINITION Abnormal uterine bleeding in the absence of organic pathology.

AETIOLOGY Hormonal influences in anovulatory and (less commonly) ovulatory cycles.

ASSOCIATIONS/RISK FACTORS Extremes of reproductive age, obesity.

EPIDEMIOLOGY Prevalence difficult to estimate, ? >10% of women (of which 20% are adolescents and 40% are >40 years).

HISTORY Commonly menorrhagia, ?IMB, ?associated dysmenorrhoea.

EXAMINATION
General: Signs of anaemia.
Abdomen/pelvis: Should be normal (diagnosis of exclusion).

PATHOLOGY/PATHOGENESIS
Anovulatory (90%): Failure of follicular development (therefore no ↑ in progesterone) leads to cystic hyperplasia of the endometrial glands with hypertrophy of the columnar epithelium (unopposed oestrogen stimulation). Shedding of this may be prolonged/ irregular.
Ovulatory: Prolonged progesterone secretion causing irregular shedding.

INVESTIGATIONS It is a diagnosis of exclusion.
Bloods: FBC (anaemia), TFTs, clotting and haematinics only if clinical suspicion of relevant pathology.
Microbiology: HVS, endocervical/Chlamydia swabs (rule out infection).
Imaging: Pelvic USS (assess endometrial thickness, fibroids, endometrial polyps etc.).
Tissue diagnosis: Pipelle biopsy/hysteroscopy in certain subgroups (rule out malignancy/ endometrial hyperplasia).
Other: Cervical smear.

MANAGEMENT
Medical: Tranexamic acid and mefenamic acid, norethisterone (day 5–26 of cycle), COCP, IUS.
Surgery: (Last resort if family is complete) hysterectomy, endometrial ablation.

COMPLICATIONS Disruption of activities of daily living, anaemia.

PROGNOSIS Majority relieved with medical treatment, but a minority require surgery (significantly reduced by advent of IUS).

Dysmenorrhoea

DEFINITION Painful menstruation.

AETIOLOGY
Primary: Occurs in the absence of pathology
Secondary: Identifiable underlying pathology.

ASSOCIATIONS/RISK FACTORS
Primary: Time period shortly after menarche.
Secondary: Endometriosis, adenomyosis, PID, pelvic congestion syndrome, menorrhagia, fibroids.

EPIDEMIOLOGY Affects 45–95% of women of reproductive age.
Primary: Commonly young girls soon after establishing menses.
Secondary: Any time after menarche, commonly in 20s or 30s.

HISTORY Spasmodic cramping lower abdominal pain, may have radiation to thighs/lower back.
Primary: Onset with menstruation or within 24 hours, resolves within 8–72 hours.
Secondary: May occur prior to and peak with onset of menstruation.

EXAMINATION
Primary: Abdominal/vaginal examination often unremarkable.
Secondary: Findings are specific to underlying cause.

PATHOLOGY/PATHOGENESIS
Primary: Prostaglandin F2α causes uterine hypercontractility and myometrial ischaemia, uterine contractions cause further ischaemia.
Secondary: Dependent on cause (also likely to be related to prostaglandins).

INVESTIGATIONS
Microbiology: HVS, endocervical/Chlamydia swabs (exclude infection).
Imaging: Pelvic USS (?fibroids, assess endometrium if associated menorrhagia).
Other: Laparoscopy (endometriosis).

MANAGEMENT
Analgesia: NSAIDS (e.g. mefenamic acid), paracetamol and codeine preparations.
Hormonal methods: COCP, progestogens, GnRH analogues (e.g. severe endometriosis).
Surgery: Laparoscopic ablation of endometriosis, hysterectomy rare (severe intractable cases if family complete).

COMPLICATIONS Limitation of activities of daily living.

PROGNOSIS Primary – excellent with simple methods; secondary – dependent on cause.

Dyspareunia

DEFINITION Pain during intercourse.

AETIOLOGY May be organic or may have psychological elements.

ASSOCIATIONS/RISK FACTORS
Superficial dyspareunia
Infection (*Candida*, *Trichomonas* etc.), atrophy (e.g. menopause, breastfeeding), vaginismus (involuntary contraction of the vaginal muscles preventing penetration), vulval vestibulitis syndrome (chronic inflammation of the vestibule with pain and erythema), dermatological disorders (e.g. lichen sclerosis, lichen planus), scarring (e.g. episiotomy), congenitally narrow hymenal ring, vaginal stenosis (e.g. postoperative), vaginal septum, sexual inexperience.

Deep dyspareunia
PID, endometriosis, chronic interstitial cystitis, fixed uterine retroversion, pelvic congestion syndrome, pelvic adhesions, ovarian cyst.

EPIDEMIOLOGY Difficult to estimate (under-reporting): >50% of women estimated to experience occasional dyspareunia, 25% may experience it regularly.

HISTORY Superficial or deep pain during or after intercourse, may have symptoms of underlying organic cause or psychosexual issues.

EXAMINATION
Abdomen: Findings related to deep causes for example masses (rare).
Vulvovaginal inspection: Evidence of infection, evidence of dermatoses, scarring, hymenal defects, anatomical abnormalities.
Vaginal: Uterine position, mobility, masses, rectovaginal/uterosacral nodules.

PATHOLOGY/PATHOGENESIS Dependent on cause.

INVESTIGATIONS
Microbiology: HVS, endocervical/Chlamydia swabs (exclude infection).
Imaging: Pelvic USS (deep dyspareunia).
Other: Diagnostic laparoscopy (endometriosis, adhesions).

MANAGEMENT Dependent on cause.
Superficial dyspareunia
Infection: Relevant antibiotics.
Dermatoses: For example lichen sclerosis may require topical steroids.
Atrophy: Topical oestrogens/HRT.
Anatomical abnormalities: Surgery.
Vulvar vestibulitis syndrome: Steroids, physiotherapy, low-dose amytriptaline, vestibulectomy.
Vaginismus: Physiotherapy/dilator therapy ± psychosexual counselling.

Deep dyspareunia
Adhesiolysis, ovarian cystectomy, treatment of endometriosis, treatment for interstitial cystitis.

COMPLICATIONS Psychosexual issues, relationship issues, complications related to organic causes.

PROGNOSIS Dependent on cause, may respond to treatment (e.g. superficial infection and atrophy). Persistent dyspareunia can be extremely difficult to manage.

Ectopic pregnancy

DEFINITION Pregnancy outside the uterus, usually in the fallopian tubes (98%) – mainly in ampulla region. Can also occur in ovary, uterus (cornua, cervix), broad ligament, and abdomen.

AETIOLOGY Damage to the fallopian tube e.g. infection, surgery, endometriosis.

ASSOCIATIONS/RISK FACTORS STI/PID, previous tubal surgery, previous ectopic pregnancy, pregnancy with IUCD/IUS *in situ*, assisted conception.

EPIDEMIOLOGY Affects 1% of pregnancies (increasing incidence related to higher rates of PID and assisted conception).

HISTORY Abdominal pain, amenorrhoea (4–10 weeks) ± PV bleeding (often scanty dark blood), shoulder tip pain (referred), dizziness (*note:* ruptured ectopic may present with circulatory collapse).

EXAMINATION
Abdomen: Tenderness ± rebound/guarding if rupture has occurred.
Vaginal: Cervical excitation, adnexal tenderness, ?adnexal mass.

PATHOLOGY/PATHOGENESIS Tubal damage interferes with tubal transport mechanisms, cilial dysfunction increases the chance of the fertilised ovum implanting in the tube.

INVESTIGATIONS
Urine: βHCG.
Bloods: FBC, clotting, X-match, serum βHCG. if diagnosis uncertain repeat after 48 hours. Levels in intrauterine pregnancy will usually double, with a sub-optimal rise in ectopic pregnancy.
USS: TVS.

MANAGEMENT All Rhesus-negative women should receive anti-RhD prophylaxis.
Conservative: Only permissible in a stable, asymptomatic patient with falling βHCG levels (tubal abortion).
Medical: Methotrexate injection – if patient clinically stable, asymptomatic, no blood in the pouch of douglas on USS, normal renal and liver function, βHCG <3000 iu/L, ectopic <4 cm in size and no FH detected.
Surgery: If patient is stable, laparoscopic salpingectomy is procedure of choice; if patient unstable or laparoscopy not possible, laparatomy. Salpingotomy may be considered in the presence of contralateral tubal disease, with increased risk of future ectopic pregnancy.

COMPLICATIONS Rupture, haemorrhage, death, tubal infertility, psychological sequelae.

PROGNOSIS Reported 5 deaths per year from ectopic pregnancy in the UK, 15% risk of ectopic in future pregnancies.

Endometriosis

DEFINITION Presence of endometrial tissue outside the uterus.

AETIOLOGY Suggested theories include: (i) retrograde menstruation (Sampson's theory), the passage of endometrial tissue through the fallopian tubes into the pelvis during menstruation; (ii) metaplasia of coelomic epithelium into endometrial glands (Meyer's theory); (iii) vascular and lymphatic dissemination; (iv) immune; (v) genetic.

ASSOCIATIONS/RISK FACTORS Nulliparity, family history, short menstrual cycle, long periods.

EPIDEMIOLOGY Affects 10–15% of women of reproductive age.

HISTORY Cyclical dysmenorrhoea (starting premenstrually and reaching peak at onset of menstruation), dyspareunia, chronic pelvic pain, infertility. Rarely symptoms of involvement of other organs/distant sites: cyclical haematuria, PR bleed, epistaxis, haemoptysis.

EXAMINATION
Vaginal: (Often unremarkable) pelvic tenderness, immobile uterus, tender uterosacral ligaments, palpable uterosacral nodules.

PATHOLOGY/PATHOGENESIS Ectopic endometrial tissue induces a chronic, inflammatory reaction. Can cause fibrosis/adhesions. Classic 'Powder-burn' or 'gun-shot' lesions seen on pelvic surfaces. On the ovary, an endometriotic cyst can form which enlarges with blood during each menstrual cycle (endometrioma/chocolate cyst).

INVESTIGATIONS
USS: Endometrioma, differential diagnosis.
Laparoscopy: Gold standard for diagnosis.

MANAGEMENT
Medical: Analgesia (NSAIDs), suppression of ovulation (COCP, progestogens, Mirena IUS, GnRH analogues).
Surgical: Laparoscopic ablation/excision of lesions, adhesiolysis, ovarian cystectomy, rarely TAH/BSO (last resort).

COMPLICATIONS Ovarian cyst accident (endometrioma), infertility, chronic pelvic pain, adhesions, sexual dysfunction.

PROGNOSIS Medical management improves symptoms in 80–90%, but recurs if treatment stopped. Symptoms subside in pregnancy and menopause.

Endometritis

DEFINITION Infection of the endometrium.

AETIOLOGY Ascending infection from lower genital tract, may occur secondary to instrumentation of the uterus.

ASSOCIATIONS/RISK FACTORS

Obstetric: Caesarean section, prolonged rupture of membranes, prolonged labour, retained products of conception, manual removal of placenta.

Gynaecological: PID/infection (Chlamydia, bacterial vaginosis, tuberculosis), instrumentation of uterus (e.g. TOP).

EPIDEMIOLOGY Incidence after vaginal delivery 1–3%, after Caesarean section 15–40%.

HISTORY Fever, abdominal pain, offensive discharge/lochia, dyspareunia.

EXAMINATION

General: Pyrexia, tachycardia.
Abdomen: Lower abdominal tenderness.
Vaginal: Offensive discharge, uterine tenderness, adnexal tenderness.

PATHOLOGY/PATHOGENESIS

Acute: Neutrophils present in endometrial glands.
Chronic: Plasma cells and lymphocytes in endometrial stroma.
Pathogens include: Gram-positive (*Staphylococcus*, *Streptococcus*), Gram-negative (*E. coli*, *Klebsiella*, *Proteus*, *Enterobacter*, *Gardnerella*, *Neisseria*), and anaerobes (*Bacteroides*).

INVESTIGATIONS

Bloods: FBC, CRP (acute infection).
Microbiology: HVS, endocervical/Chlamydia swab, blood culture.

MANAGEMENT Broad-spectrum antibiotics, surgery may be indicated if retained products of conception (after 24-hour antibiotic cover).

COMPLICATIONS PID, Asherman's syndrome, pyometra, infertility.

PROGNOSIS Ninety percent resolve after 48–72 hours with antibiotic therapy.

Fibroids

DEFINITION Benign tumours (leiomyomas) arising from myometrium.

AETIOLOGY Hormone dependent: contain large numbers of oestrogen and progesterone receptors. Enlarge in pregnancy ($\uparrow$ oestrogen) and shrink in menopause ($\downarrow$ oestrogen). Exact cause unknown.

ASSOCIATIONS/RISK FACTORS Nulliparity, family history, obesity, Afro-Caribbean race. Reduced risk: smoking, long-term hormonal contraceptive use.

EPIDEMIOLOGY Affect 30% of women of reproductive age.

HISTORY Menorrhagia, dysmenorrhoea, abdominal swelling, pressure symptoms (bowel/bladder), dyspareunia, miscarriage, infertility (*note:* often asymptomatic).

EXAMINATION
Abdomen: ?palpable pelvic mass.
Vaginal: Uterine enlargement.

PATHOLOGY/PATHOGENESIS Can be submucosal (within cavity), intramural or subserosal–round whorls of smooth muscle and connective tissue. May undergo secondary changes:
   (i)   hyaline degeneration (mucopolysaccharides deposits around muscle fibres),
   (ii) calcification (often postmenopausal),
   (iii) red degeneration (coagulative necrosis, often in pregnancy), or
   (iv) cystic change ($\pm$ liquefaction).

INVESTIGATIONS
Bloods: FBC (anaemia).
USS: TVS.
Other: Hysteroscopy (submucosal).

MANAGEMENT No treatment if asymptomatic.
Medical: Tranexamic acid (menorrhagia), mefenamic acid (dysmenorrhoea), COCP, IUS, GnRH analogues.
Surgical: Endometrial ablation, transcervical resection of fibroids (submucosal), uterine artery embolisation, myomectomy, hysterectomy.

COMPLICATIONS Anaemia (menorrhagia), miscarriage, infertility, malignant change in 0.1% (leiomyosarcoma). *In pregnancy:* red degeneration, miscarriage, malpresentation, PPH.

PROGNOSIS Ten-year recurrence rate after myomectomy 15–25% (*note:* fibroids regress and calcify after the menopause).

Gestational trophoblastic malignancy

DEFINITION Form of gestational trophoblastic disease associated with local invasion or metastasis. Includes invasive mole, choriocarcinoma, placental site trophoblastic tumour.

AETIOLOGY Abnormal chromosomal material of placental tissue. Invasive moles always follow hydatidiform mole. Choriocarcionoma may follow molar pregnancy (50%), viable pregnancy (22%), miscarriage (25%) or ectopic pregnancy (3%).

ASSOCIATIONS/RISK FACTORS Extremes of reproductive age, ethnicity (↑ in Japanese, Asians, native American Indians), previous gestational trophoblastic disease, diet (e.g. ↓ β-carotene, ↓ saturated fat).

EPIDEMIOLOGY Gestational trophoblastic malignancy follows 15–20% of complete moles and 2% of partial moles. Choriocarcinoma occurs in 2.5% of moles, in 1 per 20 000–40 000 pregnancies and 1 per 160 000 term pregnancies.

HISTORY Persistent PV bleeding, hyperemesis gravidarum, lower abdominal pain.
Lung metastasis: Haemoptysis, dyspnoea, pleuritic pain.
Cerebral metastasis: Headache, fits, blackouts.
Bladder/bowel invasion: Haematuria, PR bleed.

EXAMINATION Excessive uterine size for gestation.

PATHOLOGY/PATHOGENESIS
Invasive mole: Characteristics of hydatidiform mole, with invasion into myometrium, necrosis and haemorrhage.
Choriocarcinoma: Cytotrophoblast and syncytiotrophoblast without formed chorionic villi invade myometrium.
Placental site trophoblastic tumour: Intermediate trophoblasts infiltrate myometrium without causing tissue destruction. Contains HPL.

All metastasise widely, especially to lung, pelvic organs and brain.

INVESTIGATIONS
Bloods: Serum βhCG levels (persistently raised or rising following ERPC), FBC, LFT (liver metastases).
Imaging: Pelvic USS (snowstorm appearance, vesicles/cysts), CXR, CT chest/abdomen/pelvis, MRI brain (?metastases).

MANAGEMENT Manage in specialist centres (in UK: Charing Cross, Sheffield, Dundee).
Chemotherapy: Often includes methotrexate.
Surgical: Hysterectomy for placental site trophoblastic tumour.

COMPLICATIONS Metastasis, side-effects of chemotherapy.

PROGNOSIS Non-metastatic and low-risk metastatic disease: 100% cure rate with chemotherapy; high-risk metastatic disease: 75% cure rate.

Gestational trophoblastic disease (hydatidiform mole)

DEFINITION Benign tumour of trophoblastic tissue.

AETIOLOGY Abnormal fertilisation.

Complete moles: Diploid and paternal in origin with no fetal tissue, usually arise from duplication of haploid sperm after fertilisation of an empty ovum, or from dispermic fertilisation of an empty ovum.

Partial moles: Triploid with two sets of paternal haploid genes and one set of maternal haploid genes following dispermic fertilisation of an ovum, may contain fetal parts or fetal red blood cells.

ASSOCIATIONS/RISK FACTORS *See* Gestational trophoblastic malignancy.

EPIDEMIOLOGY Affects 1 per 1500 pregnancies (up to 1 per 200 in parts of Asia).

HISTORY PV bleeding, hyperemesis (↑ βHCG), symptoms of hyperthyroidism are rare (*note: often diagnosed by USS prior to symptoms*).

EXAMINATION Uterus larger than expected for gestational age, rarely signs of hyperthyroidism (↑βHCG mimics TSH).

PATHOLOGY/PATHOGENESIS

Macro: Grape-like appearance in complete moles, partial moles may contain recognisable fetal tissue.

Micro: Hydropic villi, atypical hyperplastic trophoblasts in complete moles, focal villi swelling and trophoblastic hyperplasia in partial moles.

INVESTIGATIONS

Bloods: βHCG grossly elevated.

Imaging: Pelvic USS (snowstorm appearance, vesicles/cysts).

MANAGEMENT

Surgical: ERPC (avoid uterotonics owing to possibility of dissemination).

Monitoring: Serial monitoring of βHCG in specialist centre (in UK: Charing Cross, Sheffield, Dundee), methotrexate if rising/stagnant βHCG levels, avoid pregnancy until 6 months of normal βHCG levels.

COMPLICATIONS Progression to malignancy (15–20% complete moles, 2–3% partial moles).

PROGNOSIS Risk of recurrence is 1–2%. After two or more molar pregnancies, recurrence risk is 17%.

Gynaecological infections – *bacterial vaginosis*

DEFINITION Overgrowth of predominantly anaerobic organisms in the vagina.

AETIOLOGY Overgrowth by anaerobic organisms replacing lactobacilli and causing an increase in vaginal pH (*note:* not sexually transmitted).

ASSOCIATIONS/RISK FACTORS Smoking, IUS/IUCD, vaginal douching.

EPIDEMIOLOGY Prevalence is 30%.

HISTORY Typically an offensive 'fishy' PV discharge, not usually associated with pain or pruritus (*note:* 50% asymptomatic).

EXAMINATION Thin white homogenous discharge adherent to vaginal wall, characteristic smell.

PATHOLOGY/PATHOGENESIS Organisms often implicated: *Gardnerella vaginalis*, *Prevotella* sp., *Mycoplasma hominis*.

INVESTIGATIONS Amsel's criteria (3 out of 4 required): (i) thin white homogenous discharge; (ii) clue cells (epithelial cells with attached bacteria) on microscopy; (iii) pH of vaginal fluid >4.5; (iv) 'fishy' odour on alkalinisation with 10% KOH.

MANAGEMENT
Medical: PO metronidazole or topical clindamycin.
Other: Avoid vaginal douching.

COMPLICATIONS Associated with increased risk of endometritis following TOP and vaginal cuff cellulitis after a vaginal hysterectomy. *In pregnancy:* associated with miscarriage, PTL, PPROM, endometritis.

PROGNOSIS 50% recurrence.

Gynaecological infections – *Candida albicans*

DEFINITION Overgrowth of naturally occurring *Candida albicans* in the vulva/vagina.

AETIOLOGY *Candida albicans* is a commensal of skin, gut and vagina (asymptomatic colonisation in 25% of women). Proliferation occurs with favourable vaginal conditions such as alkaline pH or a change in protective bacterial flora.

ASSOCIATIONS/RISK FACTORS Pregnancy, sexual activity, diabetes, immunosuppression, broad-spectrum antibiotics, vaginal douching.

EPIDEMIOLOGY Very common: >75% lifetime occurrence in women.

HISTORY Pruritus vulvae, soreness, 'cottage cheese'-like PV discharge, superficial dyspareunia, dysuria.

EXAMINATION
Speculum: Inflammation of vulva/vagina, PV discharge, white plaques may be observed on vulva and vaginal wall.

PATHOLOGY/PATHOGENESIS The yeast infects the epitheloid cells, developing spores and pseudohyphae.

INVESTIGATIONS
Microbiology: HVS.
Recurrent infections: Screen for diabetes.

MANAGEMENT
General: Cotton underwear, avoid douching.
Medical: Topical clotrimazole (pessary/cream), oral fluconazole (contraindicated in pregnancy), treat partner if recurrent thrush.

COMPLICATIONS Disruption to social and sexual life.

PROGNOSIS Good with treatment but frequent recurring attacks in 5%.

Gynaecological infections – *Chlamydia*

DEFINITION A sexually transmitted infection caused by Chlamydia trachomatis.

AETIOLOGY Transmission by sexual contact (30–40%) or vertical (50%).

ASSOCIATIONS/RISK FACTORS Multiple sexual partners, age <25 years, history of STIs, low socioeconomic status.

EPIDEMIOLOGY Most common sexually transmitted disease, affecting 1% of sexually active women aged 15–25 years.

HISTORY PV discharge, dyspareunia, IMB, PCB, abdominal pain, dysuria (*note:* asymptomatic in 75%).

EXAMINATION
Abdomen: Lower abdominal tenderness.
Speculum: Cervicitis, cervical/urethral discharge.
Vaginal: May have tenderness/cervical excitation.

PATHOLOGY/PATHOGENESIS Gram-negative intracellular bacterium infects epithelial cells of the cervix and urethra. Consists of an infectious elementary body and an intracellular reticular body. The elementary body attaches to and is taken up by epithelial cells. The intracellular reticulate body replicates by binary fission. The cell bursts releasing more infectious elementary bodies.

INVESTIGATIONS There is a national Chlamydia screening programme for under-25s.
Microbiology: Endocervical swabs, HVS, first-void urine samples (analysed with DNA amplification techniques).

MANAGEMENT
Medical: Doxycycline 100 mg 2× daily for 1 week, or single dose of azithromycin 1 g.
In pregnancy: Erythromycin/amoxicillin (tetracyclines contraindicated).
Other: Requires full STI screen and contact tracing.

COMPLICATIONS Pelvic inflammatory disease, chronic pelvic pain, infertility, ectopic pregnancy, Reiter's syndrome (arthritis, conjunctivitis, urethritis), Fitz–Hugh–Curtis syndrome (perihepatitis).
Pregnancy: PTL, PPROM, post-partum endometritis.
Vertical transmission: Neonatal conjunctivitis (35–50%), neonatal pneumonia (10–20%).

PROGNOSIS Good with prompt treatment, but many cases are asymptomatic. Longer term infection is associated with higher morbidity, especially fertility problems.

Gynaecological infections – *gonorrhoea*

DEFINITION Sexually transmitted infection caused by *Neisseria gonorrhoeae*

AETIOLOGY Transmission by sexual contact (75%) or vertical (neonatal conjunctivitis).

ASSOCIATIONS/RISK FACTORS Unprotected sexual intercourse, multiple partners, presence of other STIs, HIV, age <25 years.

EPIDEMIOLOGY Second most common sexually transmitted bacterial infection in the UK, with increasing prevalence: 22 000 cases in 2004.

HISTORY PV discharge, IMB, PCB, dysuria, dyspareunia, ?lower abdominal pain (*note:* 50% asymptomatic).

EXAMINATION
Abdomen: ?lower abdominal tenderness.
Speculum: Mucopurulent endocervical discharge, easily induced endocervical bleeding.
Vaginal: ?pelvic tenderness, cervical excitation.

PATHOLOGY/PATHOGENESIS Highly infectious Gram-negative diplococcus affects mucous membranes (e.g. urethra, endocervix, rectum, pharynx, conjunctiva), transmitted by inoculation of infected secretions from one mucosal surface to another.

INVESTIGATIONS
Microbioogy: Endocervical swab/HVS, requires full STI screen.

MANAGEMENT
Antibiotics: Cephalosporin, penicillin, tetracycline or quinolone (usually single dose).
Other: Contact tracing and treatment of partner.

COMPLICATIONS PID, chronic pelvic pain, infertility, ectopic pregnancy, conjunctivitis, Fitz–Hugh–Curtis syndrome (perihepatitis), ↑ susceptibility to HIV, disseminated disease (1–2%, may lead to fever, skin rash, arthralgia, septic arthritis, meningitis or endocarditis). *Vertical transmission:* ophthalmia neonatorum (bilateral conjunctivitis).

PROGNOSIS Cure rate is 95% with treatment.

Gynaecological infections – *human papilloma virus*

DEFINITION Infection of the vulva, vagina or cervix with the human papilloma virus (HPV).

AETIOLOGY Transmission is by physical contact or sexual contact, but occasionally vertical.

ASSOCIATIONS/RISK FACTORS Multiple sexual partners, unprotected sexual intercourse, immunosuppression, smoking.

EPIDEMIOLOGY Very common STI: 50% of sexually active adults have genital HPV.

HISTORY Genital warts on vulva, vagina, cervix and anus (*note:* often asymptomatic). Generally painless, but may itch, bleed and become inflamed.

EXAMINATION Pink/red/brown papules (single or multiple) that over time may display typical warty appearance. There are four types: small papular, 'cauliflower', keratotic, and flat papules/plaques (usually seen on cervix).

PATHOLOGY/PATHOGENESIS Double-stranded DNA virus that is highly infectious (↑ if warts present). Infects epithelial cells (skin, anogenital, respiratory) causing them to multiply abnormally. Over 100 subtypes are known. Low-risk types (6 and 11) cause benign genital warts. High-risk oncogenic types (16 and 18) are associated with CIN, VIN and VAIN. Incubation period varies from weeks to years.

INVESTIGATIONS The diagnosis is often clinical.
Histology: Biopsy of lesion.
Cytology: Can be detected on cervical smear.

MANAGEMENT
Medical: Imiquimod cream or podophyllin/trichloroacetic acid (both contraindicated in pregnancy).
Surgical: Cryotherapy, laser, electrocautery.
Prevention: HPV vaccine (aimed at subtypes 6, 11, 16, 18 to reduce incidence of genital tract cancers) as part of NHS programme.

COMPLICATIONS Cervical cancer (high-risk strains). *In the neonate:* laryngeal papillomatosis (vertical transmission).

PROGNOSIS HPV causes 3–4% of genital cancers; HPV 16 and 18 are implicated in 70% of cervical cancers.

Gynaecological infections – *syphilis*

DEFINITION Sexually transmitted infection caused by the bacterium Treponema pallidum.

AETIOLOGY Transmission is by sexual contact, blood-borne, or vertical (congenital syphilis).

ASSOCIATIONS/RISK FACTORS Unprotected sex, multiple sexual partners, HIV.

EPIDEMIOLOGY Uncommon but increasing: 2680 cases in the UK in 2007.

HISTORY
Primary syphilis
Painless but infectious lesions on skin (chancres) develop after an incubation period of 10–90 days, disappear spontaneously after 1 week.

Secondary syphilis
1 to 10 weeks after appearance of the chancre, development of macular-papular skin rash, sore throat, fever, headache, arthralgia.

Tertiary syphilis
1 to 20 years after initial infection, can develop into neurosyphilis (paresis, dementia, psychosis, epilepsy, tabes doralis), cardiovascular syphilis (aortitis, aortic regurgitation, heart failure, angina), gummatous syphilis (granulomatous lesions in skin, bone).

EXAMINATION
Primary: Painless genital chancre (papule, often ulcerated) with regional lymphadenopathy.
Secondary/tertiary: Examine skin, mucosal membranes, lymph nodes, neurological and cardiovascular systems.

PATHOLOGY/PATHOGENESIS Treponema pallidum is a spirochaete that survives only briefly outside the body. Requires direct contact with an infected part of the body for transmission. Invades abraded skin or mucous membranes and disseminates rapidly via blood or lymphatic system.

INVESTIGATIONS
Blood: RPR and VDRL, can give false positive results (e.g. with EBV, TB, lymphoma, malaria), therefore combine with TPHA and FTA-ABS which are more specific based on monoclonal antibodies and immunofluoresence.
Microbiology: Microscopy of fluid from primary/secondary lesions (with dark-field illumination).

MANAGEMENT
Antibiotics: Penicillin G (first choice) or oral tetracycline or doxycycline (contraindicated in pregnancy).
Follow-up: Clinically and serologically at 1, 2, 3, 6 and 12 months and then 6-monthly until seronegative.
Other: Contact tracing, requires full STI screen.

COMPLICATIONS Cardiovascular disease, CNS disease, Jarisch–Herxheimer reaction (febrile reaction to treatment with fever, chills, myalgia), congenital syphilis, ↑ susceptibility to HIV.

PROGNOSIS Excellent with treatment in primary or secondary syphilis.

Gynaecological infections – *toxic shock syndrome*

DEFINITION Rare but serious septicaemia caused by toxin-producing *Staphylococcus* and *Streptococcus* bacteria.

AETIOLOGY Multisystem inflammatory response to bacterial exotoxins.

ASSOCIATIONS/RISK FACTORS Tampons of higher absorbency, infrequent change of tampons, overnight tampon use.

EPIDEMIOLOGY Rare: up to 17 per 100–000 tampon users per year (average 40 cases per year in UK).

HISTORY Fever (usually >39°C), myalgia, rash, vomiting, diarrhoea, sore throat, headache.

EXAMINATION Fever, diffuse red macular rash, desquamation of palms and soles, ?shock.

PATHOLOGY/PATHOGENESIS Exotoxins (e.g. TSS toxin-1) released by *Staphylococcus* or *Streptococcus* trigger a reactive inflammatory cascade mediated by bradykinins, tumour necrosis factor and interleukins.

INVESTIGATIONS
Bloods: FBC (↑WCC, ↓platelets), U&E (impaired renal function), LFT, ↑creatinine kinase, ↑CRP.
Microbiology: HVS, blood culture, culture of tampon.

MANAGEMENT
General: Remove tampon (or other foreign object), resuscitate patient, supportive measures for organ failure (e.g. renal dialysis).
Anitbiotics: Broad-spectrum IV.

COMPLICATIONS Septic shock, multiple organ failure, DIC, ARDS, death.

PROGNOSIS Mortality is 5–15%.

Gynaecological infections – *Trichomonas vaginalis*

DEFINITION Genital infection caused by the protozoon Trichomonas vaginalis.

AETIOLOGY Transmisssion is by sexual contact.

ASSOCIATIONS/RISK FACTORS Multiple sexual partners, unprotected sexual intercourse, presence of other STIs.

EPIDEMIOLOGY Prevalence is 2–3%.

HISTORY Green/yellow (sometimes 'frothy') offensive discharge, vaginal soreness, pruritis vulvae, dysuria, dyspareunia (*note:* may be asymptomatic).

EXAMINATION

Speculum: PV discharge, vulval/vaginal erythema, 'strawberry cervix' (diffuse/patchy macular erythematous cervical lesion).

PATHOLOGY/PATHOGENESIS Flagellated protozoa that infects vaginal epithelium and proliferates when vaginal pH is >5.

INVESTIGATIONS

Microbiology: Wet mount (shows presence of flagellated protozoa), HVS, requires full STI screen.

MANAGEMENT

Antibiotics: Metronidazole.
Other: Contact tracing and treatment of partner.

COMPLICATIONS Strongly associated with the presence of other STIs, PID, infertility, ↑ transmission HIV (genital inflammation). *In pregnancy:* PTL, PPROM.

PROGNOSIS Cure rate is 90% with antibiotics.

Hyperemesis gravidarum

DEFINITION Excessive vomiting in early pregnancy associated with ketosis and dehydration.

AETIOLOGY Poorly understood, but associated with high levels of HCG.

ASSOCIATIONS/RISK FACTORS Multiple pregnancy, gestational trophoblastic disease, previous HG, ↑ BMI, nulliparity, ↓ maternal age, hyperthyroidism.

EPIDEMIOLOGY Affects 1% of pregnant women.

HISTORY Severe nausea and vomiting, anorexia, weight loss.

EXAMINATION
General: Signs of dehydration (dry mucous membranes, tachycardia, postural hypotension).

PATHOLOGY/PATHOGENESIS NA.

INVESTIGATIONS
Urine: Assess degree of ketosis, exclude UTI.
Bloods: FBC (haemoconcentration), U&E, LFTs (may be transiently disturbed), TFTs.
USS: Exclude multiple pregnancy and gestational trophoblastic disease.

MANAGEMENT Admit, rehydrate with IV normal saline or Hartmann's (dextrose solutions are contraindicated), antiemetics (cyclizine, prochlorperazine, metaclopramide), PO thiamine, consider thromboprophylaxis. *In severe cases:* prednisolone, total parenteral nutrition (rare).

COMPLICATIONS Mallory–Weiss tears, Wernicke's encephalopathy (thiamine deficiency), muscle wasting, VTE (dehydration), electrolyte disturbance, renal impairment.

PROGNOSIS Complications rare with appropriate treatment.

Infertility

DEFINITION Failure to conceive following at least one year of regular unprotected sexual intercourse.
Primary infertility: No previous pregnancy.
Secondary infertility: Previous pregnancy.

AETIOLOGY
Idiopathic (15%)
Female factor (50%): Tubal disease, anovulatory (PCOS, hypogonadotrophic hypogonadism, premature ovarian failure), endometriosis, uterine factors (anomalies, fibroids, Asherman's syndrome).
Male factor (35%): Chromosomal abnormalities, endocrine causes, drugs, irradiation, infection (STI, mumps), reproductive tract obstruction, trauma (including torsion), varicocele, ejaculatory disorders, autoimmune causes (anti-sperm antibodies), previous maldescended testes.

ASSOCIATIONS/RISK FACTORS See the aetiologies noted above. Also: smoking, alcohol, marijuana use, excess exercise, extremes of bodyweight, female age >35years.

EPIDEMIOLOGY Affects 10–15% of couples of reproductive age, incidence increases with increasing age of female partner (>30% over 35 yrs).

HISTORY Duration and type of infertility, coital frequency, menstrual history, PCOS symptoms, contraceptive history, previous STIs, medical history, surgical history, medication history, social history (alcohol, smoking).

EXAMINATION
General: BMI, signs of PCOS, signs of thyroid dysfunction, development of secondary sexual characteristics.
Speculum/vaginal: Uterine size and mobility, evidence of infection.

PATHOLOGY/PATHOGENESIS See the aetiologies noted above.

INVESTIGATIONS Couples proceeding to assisted reproduction techniques require screening for HIV, hepatitis B and C.

Males
Semen analysis (volume, pH, sperm concentration, motility, white blood cells). If abnormal, consider FSH/LH levels, karyotype, USS testes.

Females
Bloods: Day-21 progesterone (confirms ovulation), day-2 or day-3 LH/FSH (ovarian reserve), serum TFTs, testosterone, androstenedione, SHBG, prolactin, rubella immunity.
Microbiology: Screen for Chlamydia.
Imaging: USS pelvis (uterine anomalies, ovarian cysts, polyps, fibroids), HSG (tubal patentcy).
Other: Laparoscopy and dye test (tubal patency), may require hysteropscopy.

MANAGEMENT Management of identified social/environmental factors. *Unexplained*: ovulation induction with clomiphene citrate or gonadotrophins, IUI, IVF.

Male factor
May require specialist urological input. May need IUI, ICSI, IVF. If azoospermic and sperm not retrievable on testicular biopsy, counsel regarding donor sperm.

Infertility (continued)

Female factor

Anovulatory: Correction of endocrinopathies, ovulation induction, IVF. With PCOS, consider metformin, ovulation induction, laparoscopic ovarian drilling (if no reponse to ovulation induction). Counsel women with high FSH regarding use of egg donation.

Uterine factors: May require hysteroscopic management.

Tubal factors: Consider laparoscopic prodedures, often requires IVF.

Endometriosis: Should be offered surgical management of endometriosis, may require IVF.

COMPLICATIONS Psychological distress, complications of fertility interventions (OHSS, multiple pregnancy, ectopic pregnancy).

PROGNOSIS Dependent on underlying aetiology.

Intermenstrual bleeding

DEFINITION Uterine bleeding between menstrual periods.

AETIOLOGY Idiopathic, hormonal contraception (COCP/POP/IUS/IUCD), endometrial causes (polyp, cancer), cervical causes (ectropion, cervicitis, polyp, cancer), vaginal causes (atrophic vaginitis, cancer), bleeding disorders, anticoagulation, STIs.

ASSOCIATIONS/RISK FACTORS *See* sections relevant to the aetiologies noted above.

EPIDEMIOLOGY Affects 15% of menstruating women.

HISTORY Assess frequency and duration of symptoms, amount of bleeding, history of infections, contraceptive history, smear history.

EXAMINATION
Speculum: Examine vaginal walls, examine cervix (?friable, discharge, evidence of IUCD *in situ*).
Vaginal: Assess for masses, assess for cervical excitation or uterine tenderness (evidence of infection).

PATHOLOGY/PATHOGENESIS See the aetiologies noted above.

INVESTIGATIONS
Bloods: FBC (anaemia), consider clotting.
USS: Pelvis (endometrial pathology).
Microbiology: HVS, endocervical/Chlamydia swabs.
Other: Pregnancy test, cervical smear, pipelle biopsy if endometrial abnormality detected on scan.

MANAGEMENT
Medical: Consider changing contraceptive preparation.
Surgical: If evidence of endometrial abnormality on USS or persistent intramenstrual bleeding – hysteroscopy and polypectomy/endometrial biopsy.

COMPLICATIONS Dependent on cause.

PROGNOSIS Dependent on age and cause. In patients aged 20–24 presenting with IMB or PCB the risk of cervical cancer is 1 per 44 000, rising to 1 per 2400 in patients aged 45–54. Only 2% of endometrial cancers present below the age of 40 years.

Intersex disorders

DEFINITION A spectrum of disorders where an individual has a discrepancy between their male or female external genitalia and their internal genitalia or karyotype.

AETIOLOGY Several conditions exist including the following:

Congenital adrenal hyperplasia (CAH): Karyotype 46XX, with excessive production of sex steroids leading to virilisation.

Androgen insensitivity syndrome (AIS): Karyotype 46XY with failure of external genitalia to respond to androgens, leading to a female phenotype.

True hermaphroditism: Possess both ovarian and testicular tissue, usual karyotype 46XX.

ASSOCIATIONS/RISK FACTORS Family history, use of exogenous androgens in pregnancy.

EPIDEMIOLOGY

CAH: Most common intersex disorder, 1 per 15 000 (↑ prevalence in Ashkenazi Jewish and Eskimo populations).

AIS: 1 per 20 000.

True hermaphroditism: Rare, less than 10% of intersex diagnoses (↑ prevalence in certain African populations).

HISTORY Variety of presentations: ambiguous genitalia noticed at birth, neonatal electrolyte abnormalities (CAH), infertility, primary amenorrhoea, delayed puberty.

EXAMINATION Ambiguous genitalia may or may not be present.

PATHOLOGY/PATHOGENESIS

CAH: Autosomal recessive gene mutation leading to (in 95% of cases) 21-hydroxylase deficiency.

AIS: Mutation of gene encoding androgen receptor.

True hermaphroditism: Translocation of portion of Y chromosome onto X chromosome.

INVESTIGATIONS Depends on presentation, but should include karyotyping, hormone analysis (e.g. LH, FSH, testosterone, 17-hydroxyprogesterone), pelvic USS.

MANAGEMENT Dependent on underlying cause but may include hormone replacement, gender assignment, counselling, removal of gonads (risk of malignancy), surgical management of ambiguous genitalia. May require input from geneticists, paediatricians, endocrinologists, urologists, gynaecologists and psychologists.

COMPLICATIONS Electrolyte disturbance (CAH), psychological sequelae, risk of gonadal malignancy.

PROGNOSIS Long-term psychological implications.

Menopause

DEFINITION Permanent cessation of menstruation, defined as 12 months after the final period.

AETIOLOGY
Physiological: Menopause occurs due to ovarian failure associated with a dramatic decline in the quantity of oocytes and a reduction in ovarian sensitivity to gonadotrophins.
Iatrogenic: Bilateral oophorectomy, radiotherapy, chemotherapy.

ASSOCIATIONS/RISK FACTORS Increasing age, smoking, autoimmune disorders, living at high altitude, chemotherapy, radiotherapy, ovarian surgery.

EPIDEMIOLOGY Average age of menopause is 51 years in UK.

HISTORY Persistent amenorrhoea (often initial oligomenorrhoea or irregular/shortened cycles), vasomotor symptoms (hot flushes, night sweats, palpitations, headaches), urogenital symptoms (vaginal dryness, dyspareunia, frequency, dysuria, recurrent UTIs), psychological symptoms (poor concentration, lethargy, mood disturbance, reduced libido).

EXAMINATION
General: Thin, dry skin, breast tissue atrophy.
Vaginal: Atrophy, may have pelvic organ prolapse.

PATHOLOGY/PATHOGENESIS Decreased follicular activity results in increased levels of FSH/LH. Oestrogen and progesterone levels fall. Low/falling oestrogen levels are responsible for the majority of symptoms in the menopausal and perimenopausal (climacteric) periods.

INVESTIGATIONS
Bloods: ↑ FSH (>30 IU/L).

MANAGEMENT
Hormone replacement therapy
Oestrogen replacement is indicated for the relief of vasomotor symptoms. HRT should contain progesterone unless the woman has undergone hysterectomy (prevents endometrial hyperplasia). Tibolone is a synthetic steroid with weak oestrogenic, progestogenic and androgenic properties that has been used for hormone replacement. *Routes of administration:* oral, transdermal (patches), vaginal (creams, gels, pessaries), implants.

Other
SERMs, calcium supplementation and bisphosphonates are occasionally used to maintain bone health. Natural supplements containing phytoestrogens are frequently self-prescribed but do not currently carry an evidence base. Vaginal lubricants may relieve symptoms of vaginal dryness.

COMPLICATIONS The incidence of osteoporosis and coronary heart disease increases after menopause (*note:* HRT is not recommended for prevention of coronary heart disease). Depression increases during the perimenopausal period. The contribution of menopause to Alzheimer's risk is currently under investigation.

PROGNOSIS With current life expectancies in the UK, women now spend almost a third of their life in menopause.

Menorrhagia

DEFINITION Heavy, regular menstruation (>80 mL per cycle) over several consecutive cycles.

AETIOLOGY Idiopathic (DUB), anovulatory cycles, uterine causes (fibroids, polyps, infections, IUCD use, endometrial hyperplasia, endometrial cancer – rare), endocrine causes (thyroid disturbance), bleeding disorders, anticoagulation.

ASSOCIATIONS/RISK FACTORS See the aetiologies noted above.

EPIDEMIOLOGY Affects 10–20% of menstruating women, accounts for 12% of gynaecology referrals.

HISTORY Excessive menstrual bleeding: elicit duration, quantity (?passage of clots), associated dysmenorrhoea, symptoms of underlying conditions.

EXAMINATION
General: Signs of anaemia, signs of underlying conditions (e.g. thyroid dysfunction/PCOS)
Abdomen: ?palpable fibroid uterus.
Speculum: Assess any active bleeding, PV discharge.
Vaginal: Uterine size, uterine/cervical tenderness (?signs infection).

PATHOLOGY/PATHOGENESIS Dependent on aetiology.

INVESTIGATIONS
Bloods: FBC (anaemia), TFTs, clotting and haematinics only if clinical suspicion of relevant pathology.
Microbiology: HVS, endocervical/Chlamydia swabs (exclude infection).
Imaging: Pelvic USS (assess endometrial thickness, fibroids, endometrial polyps).
Tissue diagnosis: Pipelle biopsy/hysteroscopy in certain subgroups (rule out malignancy/endometrial hyperplasia).
Other: Cervical smear.

MANAGEMENT
Medical: Tranexamic acid and mefenamic acid, norethisterone (days 5–26 of cycle), COCP, IUS.
Surgery: Hysteroscopic resection of polyp/fibroids, myomectomy, endometrial ablation or ultimately hysterectomy if family is complete.

COMPLICATIONS Anaemia (10%), disruption of activities of daily living, may rarely represent malignancy.

PROGNOSIS Majority relieved with medical treatment, a minority require surgery (significantly reduced by advent of IUS).

Miscarriage

DEFINITION Pregnancy loss under 24 weeks' gestation.
Threatened miscarriage: PV bleeding with fetal heart seen.
Inevitable miscarriage: PV bleeding with open cervical os.
Incomplete miscarriage: Passage of products of conception, uterus not empty on USS.
Complete miscarriage: Passage of products of conception, uterus empty on USS.
Missed miscarriage: USS diagnosis of miscarriage in absence of symptoms.
Recurrent miscarriage (RMC): Three or more consecutive miscarriages.

AETIOLOGY Ninety percent result from chromosomal abnormalities in the embryo (commonly trisomy 16).

ASSOCIATIONS/RISK FACTORS Increasing maternal age. More than 95% of miscarriages occur in the first trimester. If RMC, consider structural abnormalities (fibroids, uterine septae), cervical incompetence (late miscarriage), medical conditions (renal disease, diabetes, SLE), clotting abnormalities (factor V Leiden, antithrombin III deficiency, primary antiphospholipid syndrome).

EPIDEMIOLOGY Affects 10–20% of recognised pregnancies.

HISTORY PV bleeding (?tissue passed), cramping abdominal pain, ?fever (infection).

EXAMINATION
General: Assess for signs of shock, ?pyrexia (infection).
Abdomen: May have mild lower abdominal tenderness.
Speculum: Assess quantity of bleeding, assess whether cervical os open (if products seen in os, remove with spongeholding forceps).
Vaginal: Uterine size, cervical dilatation, exclude ectopic (unilateral tenderness, cervical excitation, adnexal mass).

PATHOLOGY/PATHOGENESIS See aetiologies and associations/risk factors noted above.

INVESTIGATIONS
Urine: Pregnancy test.
Bloods: FBC, G&S.
USS: Pelvis (confirm miscarriage/RPOC).
RMC: Cytogenetic analysis of products of conception.
Outpatient investigation for RMC: Pelvic USS (structural abnormalities), lupus anticoagulant, antiphospholipid antibodies, anticardiolipin antibodies, consider screen for BV.

MANAGEMENT
Heavy bleeding: ABC, stabilise patient, requires surgical evacuation. Administer anti-RhD if Rhesus-negative and >12/40 or surgical evacuation.
Missed/incomplete miscarriage: Management options are conservative, medical (mifepristone/prostaglandin), surgical (ERPC).
RMC: May require low-dose aspirin/LMWH if thrombophilia identified.

COMPLICATIONS Haemorrhage, infection, complications of ERPC, psychological sequelae.

PROGNOSIS Most patients have subsequent successful pregnancies.

Pelvic inflammatory disease

DEFINITION The result of ascending infections of the genital tract (endometritis, salpingitis, tubo-ovarian abscess).

AETIOLOGY Commonly caused by STIs (often Chlamydia and gonorrhoea). May occur following instrumentation of the uterus. Other bacteria involved include anaerobes, coliforms and *Mycoplasma genitalium*.

ASSOCIATIONS/RISK FACTORS Previous STI, IUCD/IUS (within 20 days of insertion), multiple sexual partners, age <25 years, young age at first intercourse.

EPIDEMIOLOGY True incidence unknown, but accounts for 1 in 60 general practitioner consultations in women <45 years.

HISTORY May be asymptomatic, presenting with infertility, or presents as chronic pelvic pain. *Acute presentation:* bilateral lower abdominal pain, discharge PV, fever, irregular PVB, dyspareunia.

EXAMINATION
General: Signs of infection (tachycardia, fever).
Abdomen: Lower abdominal tenderness.
Speculum: PV discharge.
Vaginal: Cervical excitation, bilateral adnexal tenderness, ?adnexal mass (tubo-ovarian abscess).

PATHOLOGY/PATHOGENESIS See the aetiologies noted above.

INVESTIGATIONS
Bloods: FBC, CRP.
Microbiology: MSU, HVS, endocervical/Chlamydia swabs.
USS: ?tubo-ovarian abscess
Other: Exclude pregnancy.

MANAGEMENT
Medical: Analgesia, antibiotics based on current guidelines (may include cephalosporin, metronidazole, doxycycline). If IUCD *in situ* and no recent unprotected sexual intercourse, consider removal.
Surgical: If there is an abscess.
Other: Consider contact tracing.

COMPLICATIONS Increased risk of future ectopic pregnancy, tubal infertility in up to 50%, chronic pelvic pain.

PROGNOSIS Depends on promptness of treatment. As it is often asymptomatic, there is high fertility-related morbidity.

Polycystic ovarian syndrome (PCOS)

DEFINITION Ovarian dysfunction associated with hyperandrogenism and polycystic ovarian morphology.

AETIOLOGY Genetic basis widely implicated.

ASSOCIATIONS/RISK FACTORS Family history, obesity, insulin resistance, hypertension, autoimmune thyroid disease.

EPIDEMIOLOGY Most common endocrinopathy of women of reproductive age (5–10%).

HISTORY Anovulatory symptoms (oligomenorrhoea, amenorrhoea, infertility), hyperandrogenic symptoms (hirsuitism, acne, male-pattern baldness), weight gain.

EXAMINATION
General: BMI, BP, evidence of hyperadrogenism (hirsuitism, acne), rarely acanthosis nigricans.
Gynaecological: Often unremarkable.

PATHOLOGY/PATHOGENESIS LH and hyperinsulinaemia are thought to cause increased ovarian androgen production.

INVESTIGATIONS
Bloods: LH, FSH (↑LH:FSH ratio now not essential for diagnosis), oestradiol, prolactin, testosterone, androstenedione, SHBG (↓), TFT, GTT (↑diabetes).
Imaging: USS pelvis, polycystic ovarian morphology defined as 12 or more follicles in an ovary or ovarian volume >10 mL.

MANAGEMENT Diet, exercise (5% weight reduction can lead to resumption of ovulation), cosmetic hair removal.
Medical: Metformin, COCP including those with anti-androgenic effects (caution with obesity) or intermittent progestogens (endometrial protection), ovulation induction (for infertility).
Surgical: Laparoscopic ovarian drilling.

COMPLICATIONS Type 2 diabetes, complications in pregnancy (pre-eclampsia, gestational diabetes), endometrial carcinoma, ovarian carcinoma, increased cardiovascular risk factors.

PROGNOSIS Weight management key to successful management and mitigating long-term risks.

Postcoital bleeding

DEFINITION Vaginal bleeding occurring during or after sexual intercourse, outside of normal menstrual bleeding.

AETIOLOGY Idiopathic, cervical causes (CIN/cancer, polyps, ectropion, infection), vaginal causes (trauma, infection, atrophy, cancer), occasionally endometrial causes (polyps, cancer), pregnancy-related causes (placenta praevia).

ASSOCIATIONS/RISK FACTORS See sections relevant to the aetiologies noted above.

EPIDEMIOLOGY Point prevalence in menstruating women ranges from 0.5% to 9%.

HISTORY Elicit frequency and volume of bleeding. Also consider: smoking, previously abnormal smears, sexual history, vaginal discharge, symptoms of infection in partners.

EXAMINATION
Speculum: Note any vaginal atrophy, examine cervix for ulceration, ectropion, polyp, IUCD, discharge.

PATHOLOGY/PATHOGENESIS See sections relevant to the aetiologies noted above.

INVESTIGATIONS
Microbiology: HVS, endocervical/Chlamydia swabs.
Cervical smear: If no recent normal result.
Other: Consider USS pelvis/pipelle biopsy if persistent PCB.

MANAGEMENT Treat any identified infections.

Colposcopy: If cervix appears abnormal on speculum examination or abnormality on smear.
Hysteroscopy: If persistent PCB with normal smear/colposcopy.

COMPLICATIONS Dependent on cause.

PROGNOSIS Between 3% and 5% of women presenting with PCB are found to have cervical cancer. Of women diagnosed with cervical cancer, 6–10% originally presented with PCB.

Postmenopausal bleeding

DEFINITION PV bleeding 12 months or more after a woman's last menstrual cycle.

AETIOLOGY
Endometrial: Polyp, hyperplasia, cancer.
Vaginal: Atrophic vaginitis, local trauma from ring/shelf pessary, cancer (rare).
Cervical: Polyp, cancer.
Other: Bleeding disorders, spontaneous ovarian activity thought to play a role where no cause found.

ASSOCIATIONS/RISK FACTORS As for the aetiological factors.

EPIDEMIOLOGY Reported in up to 10% of post-menopausal women.

HISTORY One or more episodes of PV bleeding in a menopausal woman.

EXAMINATION
General: ?signs of anaemia.
Abdomen: Assess for masses.
Speculum: Assess vulva, vagina and cervix, perform pipelle endometrial biopsy.
Vaginal: Uterine size, adnexal masses.

PATHOLOGY/PATHOGENESIS See the aetiologies noted above.

INVESTIGATIONS
Bloods: FBC (anaemia).
Radiology: Pelvic USS (thickened endometrium is >4 mm in postmenopausal women).
Tissue diagnosis: Pipelle biopsy/hysteroscopy and biopsy.

MANAGEMENT Dependent on cause (see sections relevant to specific aetiologies). If no cause is found, reassure and discharge the patient.

COMPLICATIONS Dependent on cause. Complications of investigation for PMB include complications of hysteroscopy.

PROGNOSIS Most patients have no further problems, 10% of patients with PMB have endometrial cancer.

Premenstrual syndrome

DEFINITION Distressing symptoms regularly occurring during the luteal phase of each menstrual cycle, in the absence of organic disease.

AETIOLOGY Unknown, but likely to be related to cyclical effects of oestradiol and progesterone on the neurotransmitters serotonin and GABA.

ASSOCIATIONS/RISK FACTORS Obesity, lack of exercise, dietary factors, smoking, family history.

EPIDEMIOLOGY Difficult to determine: 50–90% of women are estimated to suffer from some sort of PMS, 5–10% of women have severe PMS symptoms.

HISTORY Symptom diary useful for recording nature, timing and severity of symptoms. Symptoms include mood swings, anxiety, headache, poor concentration, lack of energy, changes in appetite, disturbed sleep pattern, bloating, breast tenderness.

EXAMINATION NA.

PATHOLOGY/PATHOGENESIS See the suggested aetiology noted above.

INVESTIGATIONS
Bloods: FBC, TFT (exclude anaemia/hypothyroidism).

MANAGEMENT
Dietary and lifestyle advice: Increase exercise, vitamin B_6 supplementation up to 100 mg daily.
Medical: COCP, SSRIs (first line), IUS, GnRH analogues with add-back HRT.
Surgical: TAH + BSO (severe cases, last resort).
Other: CBT.

COMPLICATIONS Disruption of activities of daily living.

PROGNOSIS Severe PMS may constitute a long-term problem with significant psychological morbidity.

Urodynamic stress incontinence

DEFINITION Involuntary leaking of urine with increased abdominal pressure in the absence of detrusor contraction (a urodynamic diagnosis).

AETIOLOGY Pelvic floor muscle weakness (high parity, surgery), urethral sphincter damage (obesity, surgery, irradiation), increased intra-abdominal pressure (constipation, chronic cough, high parity, pelvic mass).

ASSOCIATIONS/RISK FACTORS See the aetiologies noted above.

EPIDEMIOLOGY Affects approximately 10% of women, increasing incidence with increasing age.

HISTORY Involuntary leakage of urine on exertion (stress incontinence). Symptom diary useful (frequency and severity of symptoms), may have associated symptoms (constipation, cough, concomitant urge incontinence).

EXAMINATION
Abdomen: Assess for masses.
Vaginal: May have evidence of urine leakage on coughing.
Speculum (Sim's): Observe for prolapse.

PATHOLOGY/PATHOGENESIS Caused by either damage to extrinsic sphincter mechanism (pelvic floor damage), failure of the intrinsic sphincter mechanism (poor vascularity/loss of collagen), or failure of pubovesical and pubourethral ligaments.

INVESTIGATIONS
Urine: MSU (exclude UTI).
Urodynamics: Evidence of urodynamic stress incontinence.

MANAGEMENT
Conservative: Pelvic floor exercises, biofeedback exercises.
Medical: Duloxetine (selective serotonin and noradrenaline reuptake inhibitor).
Surgical: Tension-free vaginal tape (TVT, 80–90% improvement rate), Burch colposuspension (continence rate up to 90% at one year, falling to 70% after 5 years), injectable urethral bulking agents (short-lived but low morbidity agents which can be used after failure of other procedures).

COMPLICATIONS Disruption of activities of daily living, complications of surgical procedures (including de-novo detrusor instability, bladder injury, voiding difficulty).

PROGNOSIS Can severely impact on daily life, but surgical procedures can offer significant improvement.

Uterovaginal prolapse

DEFINITION Descent of the pelvic organs.

Uterine prolapse: Prolapse of the uterus into the vagina.

Cystocele: Prolapse anterior vaginal wall involving the bladder.

Rectocele: Prolapse of the lower posterior vaginal wall involving the anterior wall of the rectum.

Enterocele: Prolapse of the upper posterior vaginal wall containing loops of small bowel.

Vault prolapse: Prolapse of the vaginal vault after hysterectomy.

AETIOLOGY Weakness of pelvic floor muscles allows descent of the pelvic organs.

ASSOCIATIONS/RISK FACTORS Increasing age, parity (vaginal deliveries > Caesarean section), menopause, obesity, pelvic surgery (including hysterectomy, bladder repair procedures), chronic cough (e.g. smoking), occupations associated with heavy lifting, high-impact sports, constipation, pelvic mass, family history, spinal cord injury/muscular atrophy.

EPIDEMIOLOGY Affects 30–50% of women aged >50 years.

HISTORY Feeling of heaviness or descent PV, back pain, recurrent UTI, dyspareunia, urinary symptoms (cystocele), constipation/faecal incontinence (rectocele).

EXAMINATION

Abdomen: Assess for masses.

Speculum (Sim's): Assess nature and degree of pelvic organ prolapse. Nomenclature: **first-degree** – descent to the introitus; **second-degree** – extends to the introitus but descends past the introitus on straining; **third-degree** – prolapse descends through the introitus.

Complete procidentia: Third-degree uterine prolapse.

PATHOLOGY/PATHOGENESIS See the aetiology noted above.

INVESTIGATIONS

Urine: MSU (exclude UTI if urinary symptoms).

Imaging: Pelvic ultrasound occasionally required if suspicion of pelvic mass.

Urodynamics: May be used to document any detrusor instability or elicit any urodynamic stress incontinence prior to surgical repair.

MANAGEMENT

Uterine prolapse

Conservative: Pelvic floor exercises, ring/shelf pessaries.

Surgical: Hysterectomy (usually vaginal, may be performed with anterior/posterior repair).

Vault prolapse

Conservative: Shelf/ring pessaries.

Surgical: Sacrospinous fixation, sacrocolpopexy.

Cystocele

Conservative: Pelvic floor exercises, ring/shelf pessaries.

Surgical: Anterior repair.

Enterocele or rectocele

Conservative: Pelvic floor exercises, ring/shelf pessaries.

Surgical: Posterior repair.

COMPLICATIONS Ulceration (from exposure of prolapse or pessaries), urinary symptoms, constipation/faecal incontinence, dyspareunia, complications of surgery. *Cystocele:* ureteric obstruction.

PROGNOSIS Recurrence rate following prolapse surgery is approximately 30%.

Procedures

Caesarean section

DEFINITION A surgical procedure by which the fetus is delivered through abdominal and uterine incisions.

INDICATIONS Whenever fetal/maternal risks from vaginal delivery exceed those of Caesarean section. Indications include:

Elective: Malpresentation, multiple pregnancy, placenta praevia, severe IUGR, infections (e.g. HIV, active primary HSV), previous classical Caesarean section (↑ scar rupture with vaginal delivery), previous anal sphincter injury, previous Caesarean section, certain maternal medical conditions.

Emergency: Fetal distress, failure to progress, maternal conditions for which delay in delivery may compromise her safety, malpresentation, placental abruption, cord prolapse, APH.

METHOD

1. **Preparation**: The patient is anaesthetized (usually spinal/epidural, occasionally GA) and placed on left tilt to prevent caval compression. An indwelling urinary catheter is inserted.
2. **Abdominal entry**: A transverse skin incision is made 2 finger-breadths above the pubic symphysis. Occasionally, a midline vertical incision is used if difficulties are envisaged (e.g. multiple fibroids). Subcutaneous tissues are divided followed by the rectus sheath. The peritoneum is identified and entered high to avoid the bladder. The urinary bladder is reflected from the lower uterine segment.
3. **Uterine entry**: More than 95% of incisions to the uterus are transverse incisions to the lower segment (↓ blood loss, ↓ postnatal morbidity, ↓ morbidity in future pregnancies). The classical (vertical) incision is used in selected cases (e.g. lower uterine segment fibroids, placenta praevia, prematurity).
4. **Delivery**: The presenting part is delivered through the incision with assistance of firm fundal pressure. Wrigley's forceps may be used. The placenta is delivered and the uterus checked to ensure the cavity is empty.
5. **Peritoneal closure**: The uterus is closed in two layers. Peritoneal closure is not currently recommended. The rectus sheath is closed. Camper's fascia is approximated if >2 cm subcutaneous fat. Skin is closed with either subcuticular sutures or staples.

ADVANTAGES Important for avoiding maternal/neonatal morbidity and mortality when used appropriately.

DISADVANTAGES See complications and prognosis noted below.

COMPLICATIONS Bleeding (± need for blood transfusion), infection, visceral damage (e.g. bladder, ureter), VTE, fetal laceration, hysterectomy rare (↑ risk with multiple previous uterine incisions, fibroids, placental site abnormalities).

PROGNOSIS Chance of future vaginal delivery with one uncomplicated previous Caesarean section: 72–76% (risk of uterine scar rupture: 22–74 per 10 000). Increased risk of placental site abnormalities in future pregnancies (0.4–0.8%). 0.4% risk of antenatal still-birth in future pregnancies.

Colposcopy

DEFINITION Diagnostic procedure obtaining a magnified view of the cervix to examine the transformation zone and detect malignant and premalignant conditions.

INDICATIONS Severe/moderate dyskaryosis, borderline change/mild dyskaryosis ×2 on smear, 3× inadequate smear, suspicious looking cervix, glandular neoplasia on smear.

METHOD
1. Patient placed in lithotomy position.
2. Cuscso's speculum used to identify cervix. Cervix examined at low power (4–6×).
3. Saline-soaked cotton wool applied and blood vessels examined under higher magnification.
4. Acetic acid (3–5%) applied to cervix. Areas of CIN appear white ('aceto-white'), possibly due to reflection from crowded nuclei. *Vasculature:* Punctation/mosaicism may be seen.
5. Schiller's test (Lugol's iodine) then applied. *Schiller negative:* normal epithelium stains dark brown (due to glycogen). *Schiller positive:* no uptake with CIN/malignancy.
6. Biopsies taken as necessary if abnormality seen.
7. Treatment may be given at this time under local anaesthetic. *Ablative techniques:* cryotherapy or cold coagulation for low-grade disease, provided the diagnosis is established with biopsy. *Excisional techniques:* for example LLETZ.

ADVANTAGES Rapid, avoids need for general anaesthetic, low risk of complications.

DISADVANTAGES Unpleasant procedure, risks related to treatment (e.g. infection/bleeding), follow-up necessary, issues regarding overtreatment of CIN I (50% regression).

COMPLICATIONS Few from colposcopy alone. With excisional treatments the main complications are bleeding and infection. Some evidence of increased cervical incompetence in future pregnancies.

PROGNOSIS Success rates after one treatment in colposcopy clinic are estimated at 85–95%.

Epidural

DEFINITION Regional anaesthesia performed by injecting anaesthetic into the epidural space.

INDICATIONS Pain relief during labour, anaesthesia for Caesarean section.

METHOD
1. Use aseptic technique.
2. Place the patient in a sitting position with flexed spine.
3. Administer local anaesthetic.
4. Introduce a Tuohy needle through the skin in the midline between the two spinous processes (normally L2 and L3). The needle should be advanced no more than 2 cm into the supraspinous ligament.
5. Remove the stylet.
6. Attach a 5 mL or 10 mL saline-filled syringe to the needle.
7. Pressure is placed on the plunger of the syringe and 'give' is felt as the needle exits the ligamentum flavum and enters the epidural space.
8. Thread a polythene catheter through the needle and leave in place (needle removed) for 'top ups'.
9. Aspiration test – no CSF or blood should be aspirated.
10. Apply a test dose.
11. Secure the catheter to the skin with transparent dressing.
12. LA (commonly bupivicaine) administered in incremental doses.
13. IV fluids started (minimise the risk of hypotension secondary to vasodilatation).

ADVANTAGES Effective pain relief, can reduce BP in hypertensive labouring women, relatively safe, 'mobile' epidurals allow women to remain mobile during labour, no ↑ risk for Caesarean section.

DISADVANTAGES Requires continuous CTG monitoring, ↑ instrumental delivery (↓ sensation for pushing).

COMPLICATIONS Failure to provide analgesia, hypotension and fetal bradycardia (reversible with correction of hypotension), urinary retention, shivering, pruritis, short-term nerve damage (1 per 5000), dural puncture 1 per 100 (headache), epidural haematoma (1 per 10 000), paralysis (1 per 100 000), epidural meningitis (1 per 3000), respiratory depression, high block (1 per 18 000).

PROGNOSIS Most women have no significant side-effects and find labour more manageable.

Episiotomy

DEFINITION A deliberate incision into the perineum to enlarge the vaginal introitus with the aim of assisting the delivery of a fetus.

INDICATIONS Predicted excessive tearing of the perineum during delivery, forceps delivery, shoulder dystocia.

METHOD The mediolateral approach is currently favoured in the UK (Figure 1).
1. Patient is informed of the procedure.
2. The perineum is infiltrated with local anaesthetic (if no epidural).
3. As fetal head crowns: operator's index and middle fingers placed inside introitus to expose anatomy and protect fetal head.
4. As perineum distended by fetal head: incision made from midline of the posterior fourchette extending at a 45° angle to the maternal right.
5. Repair is carried out after delivery as for any perineal repair.

ADVANTAGES Reduced risk of third/fourth-degree tears in selected cases, easier repair.

DISADVANTAGES Increased incidence of haemorrhage (esp. mediolateral episiotomy, possibly due to incision of bulbocavernosus and pubococcygeous muscles), midline episiotomy associated with ↑ incidence of third-degree tears.

COMPLICATIONS Bleeding, extension of episiotomy, pain, dyspareunia, infection.

PROGNOSIS Complete healing occurs over 4–6 weeks. Short-term dyspareunia common. Well conducted research on long-term effects is lacking. Occasionally corrective surgery (e.g. Fenton's procedure) required due to painful scar tissue.

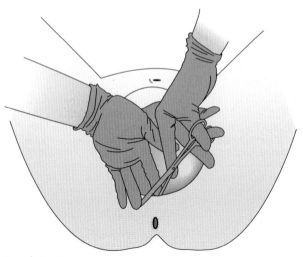

Figure 1. Episiotomy.

Evacuation of retained products of conception (ERPC)

DEFINITION Surgical procedure to remove retained products of conception after delivery of the fetus, miscarriage or termination of pregnancy.

INDICATIONS Maternal preference after miscarriage, persistent bleeding, haemodynamic instability, suspected gestational trophoblastic disease, infected products of conception (after treatment with IV antibiotics).

METHOD Vacuum aspiration is the method of choice. PO/PV prostaglandin may be administered pre-procedure for ease of operation. Widely performed under general anaesthetic in the UK although can be performed using local. Use of oxytoxics associated with reduced blood loss.
1. Bimanual examination performed to assess uterine size and position.
2. Cervix dilated if necessary (use of a uterine sound is contraindicated).
3. An appropriately sized suction catheter is selected.
4. Tissue is removed via suction aspiration and the products sent for histological examination.

ADVANTAGES Rapid, often definitive treatment.

DISADVANTAGES See complications below.

COMPLICATIONS Bleeding, infection, cervical trauma, intrauterine adhesions, incomplete removal of products, perforation of the uterus (possibly with intra-abdominal injury).

PROGNOSIS Rapid recovery, risk of perforation is about 0.5%.

External cephalic version

DEFINITION External manipulation of the fetus through the maternal abdomen to achieve cephalic presentation.

INDICATIONS Breech presentation. *Absolute contraindications:* the presence of additional indications for Caesarean section, recent APH, ruptured membranes, abnormal CTG, major uterine anomalies, multiple pregnancy. *Relative contraindications:* IUGR, pre-eclampsia, oligohydramnios, fetal anomalies, previous uterine surgery, unstable lie.

METHOD Offer from 36 weeks in nulliparous women and from 37 weeks in multiparous women (no upper limit on gestation that ECV can be performed). Can be performed in early labour.
1. Consider tocolysis ($\uparrow$ success rate): salbutamol or terbutaline IV or SC
2. Attempts at ECV are made (stop if becomes painful for the mother)
3. Monitor FH before, during and after the procedure.
4. Give anti-RhD to Rhesus-negative mothers.

ADVANTAGES Reduced Caesarean rates for breech presentation.

DISADVANTAGES Maternal discomfort, risk of complications as below.

COMPLICATIONS Placental abruption, cord accident, feto-maternal haemorrhage, fetal distress, 0.5% risk of emergency Caesarean section.

PROGNOSIS No $\uparrow$ perinatal morbidity or mortality. Success rate is 50%. Best success rates in multips, non-Caucasians, unengaged breech. Spontaneous version from cephalic presentation to breech after successful ECV is <5%.

Fetal blood sampling

DEFINITION Test performed during labour in the presence of a suspicious CTG, to detect fetal acidosis from blood obtained from the fetal scalp.

INDICATIONS CTG abnormalities (to confirm/exclude fetal hypoxia/acidosis).
Contraindications: Maternal blood-borne viruses (e.g. HIV, hepatitis B or C), known fetal or family history of bleeding disorder, preterm <34 weeks suspected chorioamnionitis.

METHOD Cervix must be at least 3 cm dilated.
1. Place patient in left lateral or lithotomy position.
2. Amniotomy is performed if required.
3. Insert an amnioscope to visualise the fetal head.
4. Fetal scalp is sprayed with ethyl chloride to cause hyperaemia.
5. A small blade is used to make a scratch on the fetal scalp.
6. A drop of fetal blood is collected in a capillary tube.
7. Sample is analysed for pH and base excess.

Interpretation of results
pH >7.25: Normal (if CTG abnormalities persist, repeat in 1 h).
pH 7.20 –7.25: Borderline (repeat in 30 minutes).
pH <7.20: Abnormal (immediate delivery indicated – emergency Caesarean section if not fully dilated, instrumental delivery if fully dilated and technically feasible).

ADVANTAGES Reduced rate of Caesarean sections compared with CTG alone.

DISADVANTAGES Maternal discomfort, especially if no regional anaesthesia in place.

COMPLICATIONS Bleeding and infection (rare).

Gynaecological laparoscopy

DEFINITION Endoscopic (keyhole) pelvic surgery.

INDICATIONS

Diagnostic: Pelvic pain, diagnosis of endometriosis, infertility (with dye test for tubal patency).

Therapeutic: Sterilisation, adhesiolysis, ovarian cystectomy, salpingectomy, ablation of endometriosis.

Major gynaecological surgery can be also be performed laparoscopically (e.g. myomectomy, hysterectomy). The clinical factors and the laparoscopic experience of the clinician will dictate the approach taken.

METHOD

1. Performed under general anaesthetic.
2. The patient is placed in a modified lithotomy position.
3. The bladder is emptied and the uterus instrumented.
4. A 1 cm vertical umbilical incision is made.
5. A Veress needle is inserted through the incision into the peritoneal cavity (pressure <8 mmHg suggests correct positioning).
6. The peritoneal cavity is insufflated with CO_2 to a pressure of 20–25 mmHg (reduced to 15 mmHg after insertion of ports).
7. A trocar is advanced through the abdominal incision to provide a port for the laparoscope.
8. A laparoscope is connected to a light source and camera, and inserted into the port. Further ports are inserted under direct vision (avoiding the inferior epigastric vessels) for surgical instruments (e.g. scissors, graspers, diathermy).
9. The patient is now placed in the Trendelenberg position.
10. Following the laparoscopic procedure, expel CO_2 from the abdomen.
11. Suture the rectus sheath at the umbilical incision, non midline port sites >7 mm and midline port sites >10 mm.
12. Close the skin.

ADVANTAGES

Compared to open surgery: Preferred cosmetic result, improved postoperative recovery, shorter hospital stay, decreased postoperative pain.

DISADVANTAGES Prolonged operation time, expense of equipment, equipment failure, ↑ training requirements for surgeons, not suitable for all patients, may require conversion to open procedure.

COMPLICATIONS Bleeding, infection, complications of general anaesthetic, VTE, damage to other organs (injury to bowel/bladder, 3 per 1000; vascular injuries, 0.2 per 1000).

PROGNOSIS Mortality is rare (3 per 100 000), 1% incidence of port site hernia.

Hysterectomy

DEFINITION Surgical removal of the uterus, may be performed with removal of the ovaries (bilateral salpingo-oophorectomy).

Total: Uterus including the cervix.
Subtotal: Uterus excluding the cervix.
Radical: Uterus, cervix, fallopian tubes, ovaries, parametrium, upper third of vagina and pelvic lymph nodes.

INDICATIONS Menorrhagia (?fibroid-related), dysmenorrhoea (uncommon), endometriosis (rare),malignancy, prolapse, intractable haemorrhage at Caesarean section (Caesarean hysterectomy)

METHOD
Abdominal hysterectomy
For malignancy, fibroids or immobile uterus (e.g. adhesions, endometriosis). Hysterectomy is performed by ligating and securing the following: round ligament, infundibulopelvic ligament (ovarian ligament with ovarian conservation), uterine artery pedicles, cardinal ligaments, utero-sacral ligaments. The vaginal vault is then closed.

Vaginal hysterectomy
Preferred route for prolapse and heavy menstrual bleeding if clinically and technically feasible. The uterus should be mobile and normally sized. Pedicles are taken in the reverse order to the abdominal method. There is lower morbidity compared to abdominal hysterectomy. With prolapse, anterior and posterior repairs of the vaginal wall can be performed at the same time.

Laparoscopically assisted vaginal hysterectomy
Ovarian and uterine pedicles are secured under laparoscopic guidance. The remainder of the procedure is performed vaginally. This enables removal of tubes and ovaries (more difficult in vaginal hysterectomy).

ADVANTAGES Treatment of conditions listed as indications.

DISADVANTAGES As per complications.

COMPLICATIONS
Immediate: Damage to other organs (e.g. ureters, bladder, bowel), haemorrhage.
Early: Infection, VTE, pelvic haematoma, urinary retention.
Late: Menopausal symptoms if ovaries removed; if ovaries conserved, 50% chance of entering menopause within 5 years, psychosexual problems.

PROGNOSIS Depends on the indication. Overall risk of serious complications following TAH for benign conditions is 4%.

Hysteroscopy

DEFINITION Visualisation of the uterine cavity with a narrow telescopic camera (hysteroscope) passed through the cervix. Hysteroscopic procedures include: transcervical resection of the endometrium, transcervical resection of fibroids, division of adhesions. It can be combined with endometrial curettage, polypectomy and retrieval of a lost intrauterine device.

INDICATIONS Investigation and treatment of abnormal bleeding or suspected intrauterine pathology. Also used to investigate infertility and pelvic pain. Contraindictions: pregnancy, current pelvic infection.

METHOD Performed either as an outpatient under local anaesthetic (diagnostic hysteroscopy only) or under general anaesthetic.
1. Patient is placed in the lithotomy position.
2. A Sims speculum is inserted and the cervix visualised.
3. Local anaesthetic is infiltrated to the cervix in the outpatient setting.
4. The cervix is dilated.
5. The hysteroscope is connected to fluids (to distend cavity), light source, and camera (to view on screen and take pictures).
6. The hysteroscope is passed through the cervix and the uterine cavity visualised.
7. Hysteroscopic procedures may be performed.

ADVANTAGES Visualisation of endometrium and histological diagnosis.

DISADVANTAGES See the complications below.

COMPLICATIONS Infection, bleeding, uterine perforation (and subsequent damage to bowel or bladder), failure to enter cavity.

PROGNOSIS Complications are rare (2 per 1000). Mortality is 3 per 100 000.

Induction of labour

DEFINITION Artificial initiation of labour.

INDICATIONS

Maternal: Diabetes (pre-existing or GDM), cardiac disease, pre-eclampsia, obstetric cholestasis, poor obstetric history, fetal death.

Fetal: Post dates (most common indication), IUGR, fetal abnormality, APH, prolonged rupture of membranes (>24 hours).

Contraindications: Previous Caesarean section, abnormal lie, placenta praevia, severe IUGR with abnormal Doppler results.

METHOD

1. Assess favourability of cervix with Bishop score (see below).
2. If BS<6, administer prostaglandin (gel, tablet or pessary).
3. Repeat 6-hourly.
4. When BS >6, perform amniotomy.
5. After amniotomy, if poor progress/contractions commence intravenous oxytocin infusion.

Bishop score (maximum score = 10)

	Scores 0	Scores 1	Scores 2
Dilatation (cm)	0	1–2	>2
Length (cm)	>2	1–2	<1
Consistency	Firm	Medium	Soft
Position of cervix	Posterior	Central	Anterior
Station of head above iliac spines (cm)	−3	−2	−1

ADVANTAGES Expedition of delivery to treat clinical indication.

DISADVANTAGES Requires continuous CTG monitoring. See complications below. Requires continuous CTG monitoring.

COMPLICATIONS Uterine hyperstimulation (and subsequent fetal compromise), failed induction (5%), cord prolapse, uterine rupture, PPH. May be more painful than spontaneous labour (↑ epidural uptake).

PROGNOSIS Dependent on various factors including indication for induction, parity and gestation.

Instrumental delivery

DEFINITION Delivery of baby vaginally with the aid of ventouse or forceps.

INDICATIONS

Fetal: Fetal distress in second stage of labour.

Maternal: Prolonged second stage, maternal exhaustion, maternal conditions that preclude pushing (e.g. cardiac disease, intracerebral aneurysm, myasthenia gravis, spinal cord disorders).

Contraindications: Suspected fetal bleeding disorders, ventouse contraindicated if preterm (<34 weeks).

METHOD

Ensure: the cervix is fully dilated, cephalic presentation, rupture membranes, <1/5 palpable abdominally, vertex at/below level of ischial spines.

If anticipate risk of failure: conduct in theatre as 'trial of instrumental delivery' with the option of proceeding to emergency Caesarean section.

1. Gain maternal consent.
2. Assess position of vertex.
3. Ensure adequate analgesia (epidural, pudendal block or perineal infiltration with local anaesthesia).
4. Place patient in lithotomy position.
5. Empty the bladder.
6. Perform instrumental delivery. The choice of instrument depends on the clinical situation and experience of the operator:

Ventouse

Kiwi cup (disposable hand-held device), metal cup (attached by tubing to suction device), or silastic cup (attached by tubing to suction device). Apply cup to flexion point of fetal vertex, check maternal tissues clear of cup, apply suction, apply traction with contractions and maternal effort.

Forceps

Wrigley's (vertex at outlet), Simpson's/Neville-Barnes (low cavity), or Kjelland's (mid cavity, rotational). Apply forceps blades, check positioning, apply traction. Requires episiotomy.

ADVANTAGES NA.

DISADVANTAGES NA.

COMPLICATIONS

Maternal: (More common with forceps delivery) perineal tears (↑ third-degree tears), cervical and vaginal lacerations, PPH.

Fetal: (More common with Ventouse extraction)

Ventouse: Cephalhaematoma (subperiosteal bleed), intracerebral haemorrhage, retinal haemorrhage, neonatal jaundice.

Forceps: Facial nerve palsies.

PROGNOSIS

Good: 80% achieve spontaneous vaginal delivery in subsequent pregnancy.

Prenatal diagnosis

DEFINITION Invasive antenatal tests to diagnose or exclude chromosomal or genetic disorders in the fetus.

INDICATIONS Demonstrated risk at antenatal screening, suspected fetal anomaly on USS, family history of inherited disorder, known carrier status for inherited disorder, previous pregnancy with chromosomal disorder, ↑ maternal age.

METHOD
Chorionic villus sampling
Performed from 10/40 to 13/40. Aseptic technique with local anaesthetic. USS-guided insertion of needle, small aspirate of placental tissue. Fetal viability confirmed and anti-RhD given to Rhesus-negative women.

Amniocentesis
Performed after 15/40. Aseptic technique with local anaesthetic. USS-guided insertion of needle, avoiding entry through placenta. Small aspirate of amniotic fluid. Fetal viability confirmed and anti-RhD given to Rhesus-negative women.

Cordocentesis
Percutaneous umbilical cord blood sampling. Performed in specialist units, when other methods inconclusive or unsuccessful.

ADVANTAGES Definitive diagnosis of chromosomal disorders. If abnormal, allows parents to decide whether to continue with pregnancy. If normal, provides reassurance. Chorionic villus sampling provides earlier diagnosis than amniocentesis.

DISADVANTAGES See complications below. Possible need for repeat procedure owing to failure of cell culture (amniocentesis 0.5%) or placental mosaicism (CVS 2%). Maternal cell contamination possible.

COMPLICATIONS Abdominal pain, miscarriage (CVS > amniocentesis), chorioamnionitis, limb abnormalities if CVS performed before 10/40.

PROGNOSIS
Risk of miscarriage: CVS 1–2%, amniocentesis 0.5–1%, cordocentesis 1–3%.

Sterilisation (female)

DEFINITION Surgical ligation or obstruction of both fallopian tubes as a permanent method of contraception.

INDICATIONS Desire for permanent contraception (after thorough counselling regarding the nature of the procedure, failure rate, risks, side-effects, irreversibility and alternative methods of contraception).

METHOD
Laparoscopy
Application of occlusive clips to each fallopian tube – most commonly Filshie clips (titanium and silicone rubber). Application of occlusive silicone rings is occasionally performed as an alternative.

Open method
For example at Caesarean section, or if laparascopy is not possible.

Pomeroy technique: Loop of fallopian tube made and tied off, loop portion of tube resected.
Parkland technique: Resection of the tube and ligation of the cut ends.

Hysteroscopy
Novel method where the tubal ostia are blocked hysteroscopically.

ADVANTAGES Permanent, reliable.

DISADVANTAGES Potentially irreversible, failure rate 1 per 200 (1% peripartum), ↑ risk of future ectopic pregnancy, risks of surgery.

COMPLICATIONS Bleeding, infection, anaesthetic complications, VTE, damage to other organs (bladder, bowel, vessels), risk of conversion to open procedure.

PROGNOSIS Failure rate as above. Successful reversal of laparoscopic sterilisation reported as 30–70%

Termination of pregnancy

DEFINITION Surgical or medical management to end a pregnancy.

INDICATIONS It is illegal to terminate a pregnancy in the UK except under specific conditions detailed in the Abortion Act 1967. These are:

A. The continuance of the pregnancy would involve risk to the life of the pregnant woman greater than if the pregnancy were terminated.

B. The termination is necessary to prevent grave permanent injury to the physical or mental health of the pregnant woman.

C. The pregnancy has not exceeded its 24th week and the continuance of the pregnancy would involve risk, greater than if the pregnancy were terminated, of injury to the physical or mental health of the pregnant woman.

D. The pregnancy has not exceeded its 24th week and the continuance of the pregnancy would involve risk, greater than if the pregnancy were terminated, of injury to the physical or mental health of the existing child(ren) of the family of the pregnant woman.

E. There is a substantial risk that if the child were born it would suffer from such physical or mental abnormalities as to be seriously handicapped.

METHOD Screening for genital tract infections should occur prior to termination or prophylactic antibiotics given afterwards. Contraception should be discussed prior to discharge. Anti-RhD is given to Rhesus-negative women if >12/40 or with surgical management.

First-trimester termination

Medical management: (Preferred for gestations <7/40, may also be used for gestations 7–9/40) oral mifepristone (antiprogesterone), followed 48 hours later by a PO/PV prostaglandin.

Surgical management: Vacuum aspiration of the uterus is performed (as described for ERPC) at gestations of 7–15/40. The cervix should be primed with PO/PV prostaglandin for gestations >10/40.

Mid-trimester termination

Usually medical as above (requiring inpatient admission). Surgical management >15/40 – known as dilatation and evacuation (D&E) – may be undertaken by a practitioner sufficiently experienced to do so.

ADVANTAGES

Medical management: Avoidance of anaesthetic and surgical complications, home or outpatient setting possible.

Surgical management: Quicker procedure, avoids pain/bleeding with medical management.

DISADVANTAGES Psychological sequelae, possible effects on fertility.

Medical management: Longer procedure, ↑ abdominal pain and PV bleeding compared to surgical management, risk of procedure failure requiring surgical management.

Surgical management: See complications below.

COMPLICATIONS

Medical management: Bleeding, failure of procedure (1–15 per 1000).

Surgical management: Bleeding, infection (10%), anaesthetic complications, cervical trauma (↑ risk cervical incompetence with late terminations), retained products of conception (2–3 per 1000), uterine perforation (4 per 1000).

PROGNOSIS Mortality (<1 per 100 000) and complications from early termination are low, increasing with later terminations.

Urodynamics

DEFINITION Investigation of the functioning of the bladder and urethra.

INDICATIONS Incontinence (mixed symptoms, failure to respond to conservative management), voiding dysfunction, prior to urogynaecological surgery.

METHOD
Uroflowmetry
Non-invasive. Identifies voiding dysfunction. Patient micturates onto a transducer. Plots a graph of flow rate against time. Normal flow curve displays a rapid rise to maximum flow rate (prolonged with reduced maximum flow rate if voiding dysfunction).

Cystometry
Bladder catheterised. Residual volume noted. Pressure transducers inserted into bladder (intravesical pressure) and rectum (abdominal pressure). Bladder filled with fluid. 'First desire to void' and 'strong desire to void' are recorded. Detrusor pressure calculated by subtracting abdominal from intravesical pressure. Provocative tests (coughing, listening to running water) are performed and any leaking is noted. Readings are plotted graphically by a computer throughout the test. The patient then voids into the flowmeter (flow rate and detrusor pressure measured simultaneously). Normal results include: residual volume <50 mL, bladder capacity 400 mL, maximum detrusor pressure <50 cmH$_2$O, absence of detrusor contraction during filling, absence of leakage or detrusor contraction on provocative testing.

Other tests
Ambulatory monitoring (longer test period of cystometry, during day-to-day activities), cystourethroscopy, videocystourethrography and electrophysiology in specialised units.

ADVANTAGES Accurate diagnosis, aids appropriate management.

DISADVANTAGES Specialised equipment and staffing needed, no diagnosis made in up to 25% of symptomatic women, sometimes poor reproducibility of findings within the same patient, invasive test, inhibiting for some patients.

COMPLICATIONS Urinary tract infection risk of 1%, urethral trauma.

PROGNOSIS NA.

Appendices

Obstetric examination

INSPECTION Note a distended uterus consistent with pregnancy. Note any abdominal asymmetry, fetal movements, striae gravidarum, linea negra, previous Caesarean section/other surgical scars.

PALPATION

Measurement of fundal height

Palpate the uterine fundus using the lateral border of the left hand. Measure fundal height from the symphysis pubis to the uterine fundus using a face-down measuring tape. The measure should be equal in centimetres to the number of gestational weeks ±2–3 cm.

Assessment of fetal lie

Palpate the lateral aspects of the uterus using both hands. *Longitudinal lie:* the fetal back feels hard and can be tracked along the length of the uterus. Fetal limbs may be felt on the opposite side as irregular protrusions (may move). A subjective assessment of fetal size and liquor volume may be made.

Palpation of the presenting part

Stand facing the patient's feet. Place both hands laterally on the lower pole of the uterus, palpating gently towards the midline (if necessary moving progressively towards the pubic bone). The head feels hard and rounded. Buttocks feel softer in breech presentation. Assess side-to-side mobility of the presenting part and the number of finger breadths palpable of the fetal head (expressed in fifths).

AUSCULTATION Auscultate the FH over the anterior shoulder. Assess its rate and regularity.

PELVIC ASSESSMENT IN LABOUR

Assessment of pelvic capacity

Assess convergence of the pelvic side walls, pubic angle, prominence of the ischial spines, diameter between the ischial spines, prominence of the sacral promontory, length of the sacrospinous ligament, and distance between the ischial tuberosities.

Cervix

Note the consistency, effacement and dilatation of the cervix (from closed to 10 cm). If dilated, assess the presence or absence of the amniotic membranes.

Station of the presenting part

Note descent of the presenting part in relation to the ischial spines (station zero).

Position of the presenting part

Assess the position of the fetal skull via palpation of the cranial sutures and localisation of the fontanelles (Figure 2). The position of the occiput is described as to whether it is anterior, posterior or lateral. In non-direct anterior or posterior positions, it is related to the maternal side (right or left). Assess for caput (swelling of the fetal scalp) and moulding (sliding of the parietal bones under each other, and of the occipital and frontal bones under the parietal bones).

Obstetric examination (continued)

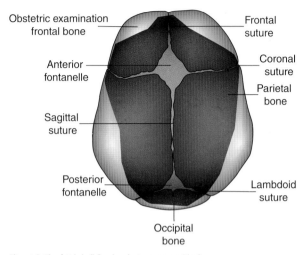

Obstetric examination frontal bone

Frontal suture

Anterior fontanelle

Coronal suture

Parietal bone

Sagittal suture

Posterior fontanelle

Lambdoid suture

Occipital bone

Figure 2 The fetal skull (landmarks to assess position)

Gynaecological examination

ABDOMINAL EXAMINATION Gynaecological examination should commence with a standard abdominal examination (using the sequence of inspection, palpation, percussion and auscultation) with particular attention to the following.

Inspection
Note any abdominal distension or visible masses (e.g. pregnancy, fibroids, tumour). Note the presence of any surgical scars.

Palpation
The left hand is used to check for pathology arising from the pelvis.

Auscultation
If the patient is pregnant, the FH can be auscultated using a hand-held Doppler instrument, from 14 to 16 weeks' gestation.

PELVIC EXAMINATION The patient lies in the dorsal position with knees flexed and thighs abducted. Gloves should be worn.

Inspection
Inspect the perineum. Note pubic hair distribution, any abnormal anatomy, erythema, discharge, vulval swellings, plaques, warts, ulcers. The patient may be asked to cough/bear down: note any incontinence or prolapse. An intact hymen precludes internal examination.

Speculum examination
A bi-valve Cusco's speculum should be warmed and lubricated. Insert the speculum sideways (direction of the blades opening laterally) in a closed position. Gently insert the speculum fully into the vagina and rotate it 90° (clasp at 12 o'clock). Gently open the blades under direct vision to visualise the cervix. If the cervix is not visualised, withdraw the speculum a few centimetres, close the blades and reposition the speculum before reopening. Inspect the vaginal walls and cervix. Note cervical ectropion, polyps/other lesions, the presence of IUCD threads. A smear, HVS or endocervical swabs may be taken at this point.

On withdrawal, retract the speculum a few centimetres in the open position prior to closing the blades (avoid trapping the cervix).

If there is prolapse, a Sim's speculum is used to visualise vaginal walls with the patient in a left lateral position with hips and knees flexed.

Bimanual examination
Insert index and middle fingers of the right hand into the vagina with palms facing upwards. Note the consistency of the cervix. Use the left hand to palpate the abdomen suprapubically. Assess the pelvic organs between the abdominal and vaginal hands. Assess the uterus for: size (described relative to size at specific weeks of gestation), position (*anteverted:* cervix points posteriorly; *retroverted:* cervix uterus points anteriorly), and mobility. Palpate the adnexa: place vaginal fingers in the lateral fornices while palpating relevant iliac fossa with the abdominal hand. Describe any masses. Note any cervical excitation (tenderness on mobilisation of the cervix).

Menstrual cycle

See Figure 3.

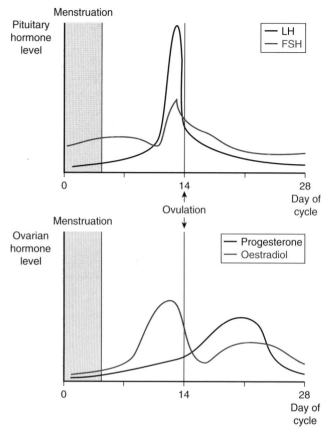

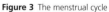

Figure 3 The menstrual cycle

Physiological changes in pregnancy

CARDIOVASCULAR Heart rate ↑ by 15 bpm. Cardiac output ↑ by 40%. Peripheral vascular resistance ↓ and blood pressure ↓ initially, followed by a rise in the third trimester.

HAEMATOLOGICAL Plasma volume ↑ by 40% (around 1.5 L) by 30 weeks. Red cell mass ↑ by only 25%, resulting in a net fall in haematocrit and subsequent physiological anaemia.

COAGULATION Coagulation factors V, VIII and X ↑. Fibrinogen ↑. Fibrinolytic activity ↓. Pregnancy is therefore a procoagulant state.

RESPIRATORY Ventilation ↑ by 40% (owing to ↑ tidal volume rather than ↑ respiratory rate). Functional residual capacity ↓ and total lung capacity ↓ (abdominal distension). No changes in FEV or PEFR.

URINARY SYSTEM Mild hydronephrosis (right > left). Renal parenchymal volume ↑ by 70% by the third trimester. Renal blood flow ↑ by 75%, leading to ↑ GFR by 50%. Plasma creatinine, urea and urate ↓. Glycosuria may occur.

ENDOCRINE SYSTEM
Adrenal glands
Aldosterone and cortisol levels ↑.

Pituitary gland
Raised oestrogen leads to increased prolactin secretion from the anterior pituitary (trophic action on breast tissue). Levels drop immediately following delivery, but remain above the normal range if breastfeeding.

Thyroid
Basal metabolic rate ↑ by up to 30%. TSH levels remain unchanged. T3 and T4 ↑, although free levels remain the same owing to increased thyroid binding proteins.

Normal mechanism of labour

As the fetus descends through the birth canal, it undergoes changes in position and attitude, in order to pass through the pelvis. In a typical (gynaecoid) pelvis, the transverse diameter (13 cm) is wider than the anteroposterior diameter (11 cm) at the pelvic inlet. The mid-cavity is circular in cross-section (12 cm diameter). At the pelvic outlet the AP diameter (13.5 cm) is wider than the transverse (11 cm).

ENGAGEMENT The fetal head enters the pelvis in the OT position. The head is engaged when the widest part of the presenting part has passed through the inlet (<2/5 palpable abdominally). This occurs prior to labour in nulliparous women (although not necessarily in multiparous women).

DESCENT Descent occurs with uterine contractions.

FLEXION As the head enters the midcavity, it flexes (chin touching chest), remaining in the OT position.

INTERNAL ROTATION As the head reaches the pelvic outlet it encounters the levator ani muscles of the pelvic floor and rotates to the OA position.

EXTENSION The head descends beyond the ischial spines. Upward pressure from the pelvic floor causes the head to extend.

CROWNING The occiput emerges from underneath the symphysis pubis and distends the vulva.

EXTERNAL ROTATION The shoulders now rotate into an oblique or frank anterior/posterior plane.

RESTITUTION The head now aligns itself with the shoulders and delivery occurs.

Antenatal care

The following is an example of a schedule of antenatal care based on the National Institute for Health and Clinical Excellence guideline, *Antenatal Care: Routine Care for the Healthy Pregnant Woman*, March 2008.

Auscultation of the fetal heart and checks for fetal presentation are not recommended unless stated, but they are often performed in clinical practice for reassurance. Further appointments/scans may be necessary in women with complications.

FIRST CONTACT WITH HEALTH PROFESSIONAL

Nutrient advice

Ensure folic acid supplements (until 12/40), avoid vitamin A supplementation, ensure adequate vitamin D intake.

Food/hygiene advice

To reduce the risk of *Listeria*, *Salmonella* and toxoplasmosis, avoid unpasteurised milk and cheese, raw/undercooked food (especially meat and eggs), paté, ripened soft cheese, unwashed vegetables. Promote handwashing prior to food preparation and after handling soil. Avoid cat litter.

Lifestyle advice

Smoking cessation, moderate exercise safe (avoid scuba diving, activities with high risk of joint stress or abdominal trauma), avoid alcohol in first trimester and recommend limit of 1–2 units per week afterwards, seatbelt advice (above and below the bump), travel advice (avoid long-haul flights, wear compression stockings with air travel).

AT BOOKING APPOINTMENT (BY 10 WEEKS)

General

Height, weight, BMI, BP, identify risk factors.

Urine

Urinalysis, MSU (screen for asymptomatic bacteruria).

Booking bloods

FBC, group and screen (identify Rhesus-negative women/red cell alloantibodies), Hb electrophoresis (haemoglobinopathies), rubella immunity, syphilis, hepatitis B, HIV.

Other

Give information regarding antenatal classes, organise dating USS at 10–14/40 weeks. Offer screening for Down's syndrome (associated with ↑ nuchal translucency, ↑HCG, ↑ inhibin A, ↓AFP, ↓ PAPP-A and ↓estriol). Options:

1. **11–14 weeks**: Combined test (NT + hCG + PAPP-A).
2. **15–20 weeks**: Double test (hCG, unconjugated estriol), triple test (hCG, unconjugated estriol, AFP) or quadruple test (hCG, unconjugated estriol, AFP, inhibin A).
3. **Both 11–14 and 15–20 weeks**: Integrated test (combined test at 11–14 weeks, followed by AFP, unconjugated estriol and inhibin A at 15–20 weeks) or serum integrated test (PAPP-A and hCG at 11–14 weeks, followed by AFP, unconjugated estriol and inhibin A at 15–20 weeks).

Concerns exist regarding the practicality of (3), so (1) and (2) are recommended depending on gestation at booking.

SUBSEQUENT CHECKS

16 weeks: BP, urinalyis, review booking tests.

18–21 weeks: Fetal anomaly USS.

25 weeks: (Nulliparous) antenatal appointment including BP, urinalysis, fundal height.

28 weeks: BP, urinalysis, fundal height, anti-RhD for Rhesus-negative women, FBC (screen for anaemia requiring iron supplementation), group and screen (red cell alloantibodies), GTT performed for women at risk of GDM.

Antenatal care (continued)

32 weeks: Further USS for women with low-lying placenta at anomaly scan.

31 weeks: (Nulliparous) BP, urinalysis, fundal height.

34 weeks: BP, urinalysis, fundal height, second dose anti-RhD for Rhesus-negative women, discuss birth plan.

36 weeks: BP, urinalysis, fundal height, fetal presentation/lie (offer ECV if breech), discuss breastfeeding and neonatal vitamin K (to prevent haemorrhagic disease of the newborn).

38 weeks: BP, urinalysis, fundal height, fetal presentation/lie.

40 weeks: (Nulliparous) BP, urinalysis, fundal height, fetal presentation/lie, can offer membrane sweep.

41 weeks: (If not delivered) BP, urinalysis, fudal height, fetal presentation/lie, offer membrane sweep, organise induction of labour within the next week.

42 weeks: Offer twice-weekly CTG and USS (maximum amniotic pool depth) for women who decline induction.

Intrapartum care

DEFINITION OF LABOUR Regular painful contractions in the presence of cervical change. *Latent phase* (variable onset and duration): <3–4 cm dilatation. *Active phase* (more rapid progressive cervical dilatation): >3–4 cm dilatation.

INITIAL ASSESSMENT
1. Check temperature, pulse, BP, urinalysis.
2. Enquire regarding SROM.
3. Monitor contractions, check FHR.
4. Abdomen: fetal presentation/lie/engagment.
5. Offer vaginal exam.

LATENT PHASE If all is well, encourage women to await the active phase at home.

ACTIVE PHASE Commence partogram. This is a graphical record of maternal and fetal observations over time. It includes: maternal vital signs, uterine activity, analgesia, other medications, fluid balance, FHR, cervical dilatation, fetal presentation and position, station of presenting part, presence of liquor and colour.

FIRST STAGE OF LABOUR Intermittent monitoring of FHR every 15 mins (for at least one minute, monitor post-contraction). Continuous CTG in those with conditions requiring it.
1. Document frequency of contractions every 30 minutes.
2. Check pulse hourly, check BP and temperature 4-hourly.
3. Offer vaginal examination 4-hourly.
4. Monitor frequency of bladder emptying.
5. Discuss pain relief options: labouring in water (if low-risk), nitrous oxide, opioids (pethidine, morphine), epidural.

SECOND STAGE OF LABOUR
1. Passive – full dilatation prior to commencement of pushing.
2. Active – pushing.

Observations as in the first stage, but monitor pulse and BP hourly. With intermittent monitoring, check FHR every 5 minutes.
If no epidural given, can commence pushing immediately. If epidural given and no fetal concerns, await 1 hour for descent of presenting part.

THIRD STAGE OF LABOUR
Active management – recommended
Routine use of uterotonics (oxytocin 10 iu IM), early clamping and cutting of the cord, controlled cord traction.

Physiological management
No routine use of uterotonic drugs, clamping of the cord only after pulsation has ceased, placenta delivered by maternal effort.

Postnatal care

CARE OF INFANT

Post delivery

1. Apgar score (*see* Neonatal resuscitation).
2. Keep baby warm and dry.
3. Encourage skin-to-skin contact.
4. Check birthweight, body temperature and head circumference within 1 h.
5. Encourage initiation of breastfeeding within 1 h.
6. Offer IM vitamin K (orally if declined).
7. Ensure passing urine, and meconium passed within first 24 h.

Within 72 hours

Full neonatal examination (often completed within 48 hours):

1. Colour, breathing, behaviour, activity, posture, tone.
2. Head circumference. Check fontanelles, palate, nose, ears, symmetry of head and facial features, assess eyes (red reflex).
3. Limbs: proportions, symmetry, no. of digits, congenital dislocation of the hip.
4. CVS: HR, murmurs, arrythmias.
5. Chest: auscultation, symmetry, signs of respiratory distress, respiratory rate.
6. Abdomen: assess for organomegaly, check umbilical cord insertion site.
7. Genitalia: exclude undescended testes in males.
8. Anus: exclude imperforate anus.
9. Spine: exclude spina bifida.
10. Note any birthmarks.

Predischarge

Offer newborn blood spot test at 5–8 days of age. Advise 6/52 check with GP for full neonatal examination and initiation of vaccination programme.

CARE OF MOTHER

After delivery

1. Check temperature, pulse, BP, uterine contraction, lochia.
2. Check placenta and membranes for condition, completeness, number of vessels.
3. Document volume of first urine void (within 6 h of delivery).
4. Repair perineal tears as soon as possible after delivery.

General

Consider thromboprophylaxis. Administer anti-RhD to non-sensitised Rhesus-negative women if baby is Rhesus-positive.

Postnatal check

Ensure observations stable, uterus well-contracted (below the level of the umbilicus), lochia normal, micturition normal, breasts non-tender, no evidence of VTE, perineum/abdominal wound healing well.

If post Caesaeran section: may eat and drink after 6 hours, remove catheter after 12–24 hours, time removal of epidural catheter with respect to LMWH (↓ risk epidural haematoma), ensure optimal management of drains if present, ensure adequate analgesia, check Hb prior to discharge, remove sutures after 5/7 (transverse incisions).

Before discharge

Offer MMR to women non-immune to rubella following birth, before discharge (avoid pregnancy for 1 month after). Advise on contraception. Advise on breast care, care of perineum/abdominal wound, umbilical cord care. Advise 6-week postnatal check with GP.

Contraception

NATURAL METHODS

1. Rhythm: avoidance of sexual intercourse during fertile period by monitoring body temperature (0.2–0.4 degree celsius rise after ovulation) and cervical secretions (spinnbarkheit during ovulation).
2. Withdrawal: removal of penis before ejaculation.
3. Lactation.
4. Persona hormone monitoring kits: measure daily urinary concentrations of hormones to detect the LH surge (precedes ovulation).

Efficacy: Poor. Pearl Index – rhythm method, 2.8/100 woman-years; persona, 6.7/100 woman-years; withdrawal, 8–17/100 woman-years.
Advantages: No drugs, cheap.
Disadvantages: Very poor efficacy, no STI protection.

BARRIER METHODS
Condom (male)
Efficacy: Pearl Index – 3.5/100 woman-years.
Advantages: STI protection, cheap, non-hormonal.
Disadvantages: Inconvenience, unreliable if used incorrectly.

Condom (female)
Efficacy: Pearl Index – 5–15/100 woman-years.
Advantages: STI protection, cheap, non-hormonal.
Disadvantages: Inconvenience, unreliable if used incorrectly.

Diaphragm.cap (female)
Efficacy: Pearl index – 2/100 woman-years.
Advantages: STI protection, cheap, non-hormonal.
Disadvantages: Less effective if >3.5 kg weight change, annual fitting check, inconvenience.

COMBINED ORAL CONTRACEPTIVE PILL Suppresses ovulation by inhibiting cyclical LH and FSH, renders endometrium inhospitable, thickens cervical mucus.
Efficacy: 0.16/100 woman-years
Advantages: Highly effective, ↓ mennorhagia, dysmenorrhoea, functional ovarian cysts, benign breast disease, fibroids, endometrial and ovarian cancer.
Disadvantages: No STI protection, not effective if poor compliance. *Side-effects:* headache, nausea, breast tenderness, weight gain, ↑ risk of VTE (5 per 100 000 non-users, 12 per 100 000 second-generation COCP (levonorgestrel), 25 per 100 000 third-generation COCP (desogestrel or gestodene), 60 per 100 000 pregnancy)
Contraindications: History of VTE, CVA, MI, active liver disease, severe inflammatory bowel disease, focal migraine, pregnancy, breastfeeding, smoker >35 years old, cardiovascular risk factors.

Advice
Start packet the first day of menstruation (no additional contraception required). Take daily for 21 days, then 7-day break (withdrawal bleed). Need to take within 12-hour window. Can take up to three packets back-to-back (tri-cycling). Extra contraception needed if taking certain antibiotics, taking enzyme-inducing drugs, not commenced on first day of period, missed pill (7-day rule).

PROGESTERONE-ONLY PILL Thickens cervical mucus, renders endometrium inhospitable, decreases tubal motility, inhibits ovulation in 40%.
Efficacy: 0.3–4/100 woman-years.
Advantages: Highly effective, ↓ menorrhagia, dysmenorrhoea, not contraindicated during breastfeeding, can be used in smokers/history VTE.

Contraception (continued)

Disadvantages: No STI protection, irregular bleeding, weight gain, headache, ↑ risk of ectopic pregnancy if contraceptive failure, ↑ functional ovarian cysts, must be taken at the same time each day (cerazette has 12-hour window)

Advice
Start packet on the first day of menstruation. Take continuously with no break.

DEPOT PROGESTERONE Suppresses ovulation. Also acts on cervical mucous and endometrium. Amenorrhoea common. Consists of 3-monthly progesterone injection (medroxy-progesterone acetate 120 mg).
Efficacy: Pearl Index – <1/100 woman-years.
Advantages: Good if problems with compliance, not contraindicated during breastfeeding, can be used in smokers/history VTE.
Disadvantages: As for progesterone-only pills, plus delayed return to fertility after cessation, long-term use associated with osteoporosis.

IMPLANT Suppresses ovulation. Also acts on cervical mucous and endometrium. Implanon® (68 mg etonogestrel) lasts for 3 years.
Efficacy: Pearl Index – <1/100 woman-years.
Advantages: Good if problems with compliance, ↓ dysmenorrhoea, not contraindicated during breastfeeding, can be used in smokers/history VTE.
Disadvantages: As for progesterone-only pills.

COPPER IUCD Prevents implantation. Lasts for 5–8 years.
Efficacy: Pearl Index – 1–5/100 woman-years.
Advantages: Good if problems with compliance, no hormonal side-effects.
Disadvantages: Requires small procedure to insert, risk of perforation, risk of expulsion, risk of ectopic pregnancy if contraceptive failure, no STI protection, risk of PID in first 20 days, irregular/heavy bleeding.

IUS (MIRENA®) Coil containing 52 mg levonorgestrel. Lasts for 5 years.
Efficacy: Pearl Index – <1/100 woman-years.
Advantages: Good if problems with compliance, improved menstrual symptoms, can use if breastfeeding
Disadvantages: As for progesterone-only pills, plus requires small procedure to insert, risk or perforation, risk of expulsion, risk of ectopic pregnancy if contraceptive failure, no STI protection, risk of PID in first 20 days, some women experience irregular bleeding.

VAGINAL RING Contains oestrogen and progestogen. Inserted into the vagina, removed after 3 weeks for a 1-week period to allow a withdrawal bleed. Efficacy is comparable to the COCP.

STERILISATION See Procedures section.

EMERGENCY CONTRACEPTION Levonorgestrel 1.5 mg within 72 hours of unprotected sexual intercourse (taken within 24 h prevents 95% of pregnancies). Copper coil within 5 days of unprotected sexual intercourse or 5 days of ovulation date (may require antibiotic cover).
Disadvantages: Decreasing efficacy with increasing time since unprotected intercourse, risk of PID with IUCD insertion, ↑ risk of ectopic if pregnancy occurs.

Cardiotocography (CTG)

DEFINITION Continuous electronic monitoring of the fetal heart and uterine activity.

METHOD
1. Fetal heart rate is monitored using Doppler ultrasound. The transducer is applied to the abdomen over the anterior shoulder. *Note:* FSE may also be used if monitoring difficult abdominally, provided no suspected clotting abnormality and no maternal blood-borne viruses.
2. External pressure transducer is applied to the uterine fundus to monitor uterine activity.

Baseline heart rate
Controlled by sympathetic (↑ FHR) and parasympathetic (↓ FHR) activity and fetal maturity (↑ maturity – ↑ vagal tone). Also controlled by chemoreceptors and baroreceptors in the aortic arch.
Reassuring: 110–150 bpm.
Non reassuring: 100–109 bpm or 161–180 bpm.
Abnormal: <100 bpm or >180 bpm.

Causes of baseline tachycardia: Maternal tachycardia, maternal pyrexia, ↑ fetal movements, severe hypoxia, infection (chorioamnionitis).
Causes of baseline bradycardia: Normal in postmature fetuses, certain cardiac abnormalities/drugs.

Beat to beat variability
Normally 5–15 bpm.
Variability is the result of constant interaction between the above regulatory factors (denotes intact nervous pathway). *Decreased:* extremely preterm fetuses, fetal sleep pattern (normal for period of 40 mins), drugs (e.g. pethidine), severe hypoxia.
Reassuring: ≥5 bpm.
Non reassuring: <5 bpm for more than 40 minutes.
Abnormal: <5 bpm for 90 minutes.

Accelerations
An increase in the FHR of at least 15 beats for at least 15 seconds.
Occurs with fetal movement or uterine contractions (interaction of the parasympathetic/sympathetic nervous system due to ↑ metabolic demands).
Reassuring: Should be present (reactive CTG).
Non reassuring: Absence of accelerations (although significance uncertain).

Decelerations
A decrease in the FHR of at least 15 beats for at least 15 seconds.
Prolonged: Lasting >2 minutes.
Bradycardia: Lasting >3 minutes.

Reassuring: None.
Non reassuring: Typical variable decelerations with >50% of contractions for >90 min *or* 1× prolonged deceleration.
Abnormal: Atypical variable decelerations with >50% of contractions *or* late decelerations for >30 min *or* bradycardia.

Classification of decelerations
Early
Onset with and recovery by the end of a contraction. Caused by fetal head compression (↑ parasympathetic stimulation). Not associated with fetal compromise. May be alleviated by change in maternal position.

Cardiotocography (CTG) (continued)

Late

Nadir occurs >15 s after the peak of the contraction. Caused by decreased uterine blood flow causing deoxygenation. Detected by aortic arch chemoreceptors leading to ↑ parasympathetic stimulation (delayed by the time it takes for blood to circulate to the aortic arch). Associated with fetal hypoxia. Necessitates FBS.

Variable

Variable in shape and relation to uterine contractions. Accelerations often occur before and after giving a classical 'M' shape.

Typical: Classic 'M' shape.

Atypical: Slow return to baseline, ↓ variability within deceleration, one-sided acceleration, overshoot (persistence of secondary acceleration), ↓ baseline post-deceleration, biphasic deceleration.

Occur due to cord compression. *Vein compression:* ↓ venous return and arterial pressure leads to ↑ sympathetic activity and fetal tachycardia to maintain BP. *Compression of arteries:* ↑ BP increases leads to ↑ parasympathetic activity (↓ FHR). *Compression of arteries relieved:* hypotension recurs causing a reactive tachycardia (returns to baseline when venous flow normalises). May be relieved by maternal position change. If persistent requires FBS.

Classification of ctgs

Reassuring: *All four* features reassuring

Suspicious: *One* feature non-reassuring

Non reassuring: *At least two* features non reassuring or *at least one* abnormal.

Neonatal resuscitation

APGAR SCORE Observations are carried out at 1 and 5 minutes of life to indicate condition at birth. A low one-minute score indicates medical attention needed (*note:* resuscitation should not be delayed in neonates clearly needing attention earlier).

	Score		
	0	**1**	**2**
Heart rate	0	<100 bpm	>100 bpm
Breathing	Apnoeic	Irregular	Good
Colour	White	Blue	Pink
Muscle tone	Floppy	Some movement	Active
Reflex response	Nil	Grimace	Cough or cry

Scores: ≥7 normal, 3–6 primary apnoea, >3 terminal apnoea.

ASSESSMENT Assessment of the neonate should occur in the first 30 seconds and be carried out frequently during resuscitation:

Well/vigorous: Pink, good tone, good respiratory effort, heart rate >100 bpm

Primary apnoea (needs medical attention): Cyanosed, poor tone, poor respiratory effort ± heart rate <100 bpm.

Terminal apnoea (requires full intensive resuscitation): Pale, floppy, poor respiratory effort, heart beat <60 bpm or absent.

INITIAL ATTENTION

1. Most neonates needing resuscitation will respond to lung inflation. Very few require chest compression, even fewer require drugs (poor prognosis).
2. Removing meconium from airways is not recommended except in unresponsive babies born through thick meconium (under direct vision).
3. Ensure warmth throughout resuscitation (lose heat very quickly).

SEQUENCE OF RESUSCITATION

1. Dry and stimulate baby, wrap in dry towel, place under radiant heater.
2. Preterm <30 weeks: place in food-grade plastic wrapping, with face uncovered, without drying.
3. Assess colour, tone, breathing and heart rate.

Airway

Place baby on back with head in neutral position (consider jaw thrust).

Breathing

If inadequate breathing after 90 seconds:

1. Five inflation breaths each of pressure 30 cmH$_2$O for 2–3 seconds (lungs initially filled with fluid).
2. If HR >100 bpm but no breathing, continue inflation (rate 30–40/min) until spontaneous breaths.
3. If HR <60 bpm, check lungs inflating with adequate chest movement. (If inadequate inflation check head position, consider obstruction in oropharynx - remove under direct vision if necessary, consider tracheal intubation).

Neonatal resuscitation (continued)
Circulation
If HR<60 bpm following adequate inflation breaths, commence chest compression. Hold chest in both hands with fingers over the spine and thumbs on the lower 1/3 of the sternum below an imaginary line joining the nipples. Compress chest by 1/3 with thumbs (rate of 120/min, ratio *three* compressions for each inflation).

Drugs
Use an umbilical catheter (*note:* intraosseus route may be used).
Adrenaline (1 : 10 000): 10 μg/kg (0.1 mL/kg) up to 30 μg/kg (0.3 mL/kg).
Sodium bicarbonate: 1–2 mmol bicarbonate/kg (2–4 mL/kg of 4.2% bicarbonate solution).
Dextrose: 250 mg/kg (2.5 mL/kg of 10% dextrose).

Note: If significant volume loss is suspected, give 10 mg/kg 0.9% saline bolus over 10-20 seconds.